Effects of and Interventions for Childhood Trauma from Infancy Through Adolescence
Pain Unspeakable

Sandra B. Hutchison, LCSW, BCETS

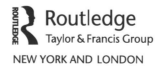
Routledge
Taylor & Francis Group

NEW YORK AND LONDON

First published 2005 by The Haworth Press, Inc.

This edition published 2011 by Routledge
605 Third Avenue, New York, NY 10017
2 Park Square, Milton Park, Abingdon, Oxon OX

Routledge is an imprint of the Taylor & Francis (

PUBLISHER'S NOTE
Identities and circumstances of individuals discussed in
confidentiality.

Cover design by Kerry E. Mack.

Library of Congress Cataloging-

Hutchison, Sandra B.
    Effects of and interventions for childhood trauma
unspeakable / Sandra B. Hutchison.
        p. cm.
    Includes bibliographical references and index.
    ISBN 0-7890-0856-4 (hard : alk. paper)—ISBN 0-7
    1. Child analysis. 2. Psychic trauma in children. I. T
RJ504.2.H885 2004
618.92'8521—dc22

ISBN 13: 978-0-7890-2428-2 (pbk)

DOI: 10.4324/9780203048030

To my loving husband, Charles,
and my two adorable children, Aba and Nana,
for bringing such joy and purpose into my life
and inspiring me beyond limits

Sandra B. Hutchison, LCSW, BCETS
pendent consultant in Charlotte, North
fied and a diplomate of the American ⌐
matic Stress and is listed in the Acad⌐
She currently practices at a day treatm⌐
emotional and behavioral disorders. ⌐
censed clinical social worker for the
Georgia, and as Lead Clinician and C⌐
vices at the Bristol Bay Area Health ⌐
Department in Dillingham, Alaska.

For over fifteen years, Ms. Hutchiso⌐
have survived numerous traumatic eve⌐
ual abuse, rape, family violence, natura⌐
family member. She has conducted pre⌐
child mental health and provided consu⌐
as schools, child care centers, hospital⌐
agencies, and medical facilities.

Ms. Hutchison has also served as a ⌐
team in rural Alaska. She has respond⌐
dents involving children, such as the ra⌐
cent which left a police officer dead, a
very young children, the drowning of
holds certificates of training in disaste⌐
the American Red Cross and in corp⌐
threat of violence consultation from
tional, Inc., in Atlanta, Georgia.

Ms. Hutchison majored in child stud⌐
ment of Child Development at Tufts U⌐
degrees in both child study and mental
She then received her MSS in clinical ⌐
College Graduate School of Social Wo⌐

CONTENTS

Foreword

For those who have had the misfortune (privilege) of being first-line responders to a major traumatic event affecting children, this book is an excellent summary of the thoughts, fears, expectations, and lessons learned in the process. Reading the book, I could not help wishing it had been published before August 1998, when terrorists exploded a one-ton bomb at the U.S. Embassy in Nairobi on the very morning of the National Music Festival. Several thousand school children were within a block of the epicenter of the explosion. Beyond the physical injuries suffered by many, half the children exhibited symptoms of acute stress disorder (boys more than girls, younger more than older), and many went on to develop full-blown PTSD. Their reactions were very similar to the children of Oklahoma and later of New York City. In a sense, this similarity is to be expected when children's blood is shed by the hands of terrorists, men and women in pursuit of goals beyond the comprehension of the victims.

By its very nature, trauma to children is unexpected, unnatural, but increasingly common. It traumatizes and confuses both the child and the adult responders to the aftermath. The pain of watching children in trauma is therefore magnified by the feelings of despair, hopelessness, and inadequacy that engulf adults as they grapple with both the causes and consequences of the traumatic events. The adult in these situations must not only deal with each child's needs but must at the same time deal with his or her own fear and insecurity, which he or she mostly tries to hide from the children. In this respect, the pain of the adult responder is also unspeakable. To this extent, it often (if not acknowledged) impedes the efficiency of the adult responding to the children's needs.

This book is a true and valuable addition to the knowledge base in the advancement of the tools of intervention for those on the front line of response. The fact that it addresses all cadre of mental health responders makes it even more appropriate and relevant, because psychologists, psychiatrists, social workers, and to some extent teachers will have a common instrument of reference in their hour of greatest

need. In it, I see an interesting additior
teams respond to the aftermath of the d
an intact team as they discuss the varic
ment is ideal for this type of approach.

Beyond its easy readability, this is a
vance to many other experts likely to be
sues in a commonsense and practical m

Children (in their innocence) are perl
common denominators across cultures,
described in this text have a relevance ac
adults may not. The chapter titled Unde
Trauma speaks for the children in genera
on developmental considerations and
matic incidents. Those who have practic
identify with the relevance of these chap
children seem to need the same level of
That children in Africa are traumatize
wars makes them victims similar to the
bodia. Their needs, fears, and responses
cal. The effects of September 11, 2001
children in similar ways to earlier traum
bassy bombing.

The lessons from the chapter on in
nance with those who have past firsthanc
and it must be taken seriously by those
needing to implement similar interver
cance is the need to take services to the
one assured of the maintenance of the ch
ing the critical days and weeks after the
a sense of normalcy is critical to the recc
be both a friend and foe, and special an
tory, as is the requirement for maintenan
out the response period, achieved best b

This book comes out at a time of inc
ing children. Because its approach is cu
value and utility across national and int

President, African

Acknowledgments

I wish to acknowledge the people who have helped to make this book possible, including my family and those professionals who have shared their insights, expertise, joys, and heartaches over the years.

My husband, Dr. Charles Hutchison, has been very supportive and inspirational. I thank him for working overtime to help care for our four-year-old son, Nana, and our eight-year-old daughter, Aba, by performing various household chores, helping with meals, giving baths, etc. He juggled all these tasks, in addition to teaching full-time at a university, while I worked diligently to complete this book. My children have been a blessing as well, and I am thankful to them for being the joy in my life.

Professionally speaking, I would like to thank Dr. David Elkind, who was my mentor in college and who shared his words of wisdom; Dr. Martin Zelin, who was my academic advisor and the first to introduce me to the field of clinical social work; Dr. David Harder, who informed me that being an extrovert was not a requirement for entering the profession; and Dr. Marcia Martin, who inspired me to work with children.

I would also like to acknowledge my colleagues: Yvette Pack-Logan, who has been a dear and supportive friend ever since graduate school; Joan Ribich, who agreed to hire a "city girl," such as myself, to provide counseling services in remote Eskimo villages in below-zero temperatures; and Don Cline, for his training in debriefing techniques and his sense of humor when needed.

Introduction

> Every adult, whether he is a follower or a leader, a member of a mass or of an elite, was once a child. He was once small. (Erikson, 1950, p. 360)

Imagine the world of children. Children start out their lives dependent on adults for their care and sustenance. They begin their growth and development in the comfort and warmth of their mothers' wombs, where all their needs are met. They are unaware of the lives that await them on the outside.

Eventually these children undergo the rather stressful process of birth. As they are brought forth into the world, they, along with their parents, experience a rigorous test of physical and emotional endurance that no words can explain. For the first time, these new beings are able to see other people and objects, hear many different sounds, feel various textures, and taste their mothers' milk. As their needs are met, they begin to develop trust in their new environment and find that life on the outside is tolerable after all.

The time comes, however, for children and their parents to "separate" for continued growth to take place. Children transition from home to the school environment and are entrusted to additional adult caregivers—those who have courageously stepped up to the task of caring for the world's children.

The role of caregivers (educators, counselors, health care professionals, etc.) is a courageous one indeed, and it is multifaceted. It is a role that involves teaching children to exercise their full potential; counseling children to believe that they even have potential to begin with; healing their pains, both emotional and physical; and protecting them from the very elements that afflict them.

Those firsts will take place: a scraped knee or elbow, a hurt feeling, a push and a shove, a "bad" report card, teasing remarks, a losing game, or rejection from a friend. Both parents and caregivers try their best to alleviate these trials of childhood.

Some pain, however, cannot be alle
couragement and a hug, nor can it be
wounds are far too deep, the memories
scars ever visible. This is the kind of pa
regress to a state of utter helplessness a
cause a gregarious, self-assured adoles
drawn and uncommunicative. This ty
only by a traumatic incident that coulc
effects of a hurricane, the horror of sex
or the dangerous path of gunfire.

The traumatic suffering of children
about, nor was it easy to write about.
young, innocent, defenseless children w
to be sold by their "pimps," or having ;
into their hands and being forced to kil
the name of war.

Imagine children being savagely be
brought them into the world; children
face in a river following a natural disa
tage by their own classmates armed wit.
dren feeling so helpless and depressed th
lives.

Does this sound melodramatic? Perh
ries of countless children throughout th
selves face to face with trauma. Caregiv
reach out to these children. It can mean
to hold onto, warm blankets to wrap the
ear, or the reassurance that you care an
mean offering them nutritious food to e
line number to call, family support, fa
education, advocacy, supportive coun
medical treatment.

As caregivers, you have been charged
suring the protection and harmonious
who come under your care, especially
only your presence but also your readir
world to children who may have lost
them—parents, siblings, homes, comm
nity, self-esteem, innocence, and rights

the field of mental health, education, advocacy, or health care, caregivers share one common goal: to help create a safe place for all children to learn and grow. It is my hope that this book will be useful in that endeavor.

I have attempted to note traumatic incidents, statistical information, and research that have taken place in the United States as well as in other regions of the world. Cultural considerations are also mentioned throughout the book. It is important to adopt a global perspective in the work that we do, especially as it relates to trauma.

Approximately 95,000 foreigners arrive in the United States every day. About 3,000 of these daily arrivals are immigrants or refugees who have been invited to become permanent residents of the United States. The U.S. population is projected to reach 409 million in 2050. Hispanics are, currently, the largest ethnic minority group in the United States and are expected to make up 25 percent of the population in 2050. Asians and Pacific Islanders will make up 10 percent of the population in that time period (Martin and Midgley, 2003). A rapidly growing Arab population, a sizable Jewish population, and numerous other ethnic groups will add to the cultural diversity in the United States (Pollard and O'Hare, 1999).

By the middle of the twenty-first century, ethnic minorities will compose nearly 50 percent of all Americans (O'Hare, 1992). The United States is thus transforming from a predominately white population dominated by Western culture to a society composed of diverse racial and ethnic minorities (O'Hare, 1992).

Ethnic minority children are the largest-growing segment of the U.S. population (Aponte and Wohl, 2000). As a result, the racial and ethnic makeup of the nation's school population is undergoing a profound change. Classrooms are continuously being filled with children who speak, eat, dress, and behave in ways that differ from mainstream American culture. Many will enter the United States traumatized due to the very reasons for leaving their countries (e.g., political unrest, terrorism, war, famine, oppression, natural disaster, and other hardships) and the means by which they had to leave (e.g., seeing family members shot while fleeing or undergoing brutal attacks by bandits, etc.).

For example, various types of traumatized populations emerged during the 1990-1991 Persian Gulf War. Non-Kuwaiti Arabs, including Lebanese and Palestinians, were displaced from Kuwait due to

the war. Some refugees were intact far
infants who had to leave the country
(Abudabbeh, 1994). According to Abu
had emigrated from Lebanon or the
ported to be reliving early traumas thro
problems.

The majority of new immigrants con
the third world—the underdeveloped nat
na, 1996). Many refugees from Cuba a
homes by either boat or plane to esc
death situations. Those who survived
fered from post-traumatic stress disorc
hypervigilance, nightmares, flashback:
(Gopaul-McNicol and Brice-Baker, 19

The Southeast Asian refugee exodu
of Vietnam, Cambodia, and Laos fror
1980s is one of the largest refugee
Many Vietnamese immigrated to the U
lapse of Vietnam in 1975, or escaped as
1970s (Kinzie et al., 1990). The Camb
were also displaced by the Vietnam Wa
separation of families, and witnessing
riences among all Southeast Asian re
1990).

Cambodian refugee children who in
were separated from their families, enc
tion, and witnessed many deaths during
their traumatic experiences and accomp
them (Kinzie et al., 1986).

In a study of the effects of trauma or
gees, Sack and colleagues (1986) pres
high school student whose memories o
tion of 200 people were triggered durir
movie.

Adults who are concerned with
must have a clear understanding of
children do not drop their culture
day begins. The child brings to th
patterns of his home. (Landau, Eps

Apparently, many Cambodian refugees continued to experience severe PTSD and related symptoms four to six years after their arrival in the United States (Carlson and Rosser-Hogan, 1991). As caregivers, it is important that we are knowledgeable of the traumatic incidents that occur in the United States, as well as in various regions of the world. We also need to know how trauma manifests itself across cultures, and we must use culturally sensitive approaches to intervention. We cannot operate as if we are unfazed by global events. Whatever happens globally does have a tendency to show up in the United States—in our communities, schools, and treatment facilities—and it is crucial that we prepare ourselves to respond appropriately.

Chapter 1 of this book depicts the many faces of trauma. It features actual accounts of traumatic incidents throughout the world, such as threats or acts of violence, school bus accidents, fires, and natural disasters. I have discussed incidents that are known to have the most devastating impact on large groups of children. The kinds of incidents that traumatize children, however, are not limited to those mentioned in this section.

Chapter 2 applies Erikson's psychosocial stages of ego development to the understanding of children's reactions to traumatic incidents. Memory development, the experience of fear, and the conceptual understanding of death at the various age levels are addressed, as are cultural considerations.

Chapter 3 describes how children of different age groups respond to traumatic incidents. A review of the research on PTSD and stress-response-related symptoms, such as intrusive imagery, sleep disturbances, somatic complaints, and avoidant responses, is also provided. Specific reactions to terrorism and war trauma, as well as cultural considerations, are addressed.

Chapter 4 provides brief descriptions of the various treatment modalities applied to children who suffer from posttraumatic stress. Cultural considerations are also addressed and case examples are presented.

Chapter 5 is geared toward those who work with children in school settings and explains how to establish a trauma response team. A curtailed description is given of the various functions and responsibilities of team members and faculty, including rumor control, meeting

with the media, preparing to meet with
faculty group debriefings, and facilitati

The Resources section suggests read
various traumatic incidents. It also list
names of organizations that can provid

Chapter 1

Understanding the Many Faces
of Trauma

At the instant a terrible event strikes, what does a child do? Does
he freeze, run, vomit, defecate, lose his temper, shriek, cry, or
become mute? Usually, of course, there are no photographs of a
traumatic event to consult after the fact. (Terr, 1990, p. 32)

A DEFINITION OF TRAUMA

Many people experience stress in their lives as a result of life
changes, such as a loss of job, change of school or neighborhood,
family conflict, or new addition to the family. Stress is an unavoidable
and expected occurrence in one's lifetime. Fortunately, we develop
ways of coping and are able to move on to the next phase of our lives.

Children are no strangers to stressful life events. They experience
stress as early as the birth process itself and maybe even in the womb.
Nevertheless, most children are able to survive and flourish.

Terr (1990) differentiates life stresses from psychological trauma,
even though the two terms are often used interchangeably. She de-
fines stress as an expectable occurrence in an ordinary lifetime. Trauma
is not. According to Terr (1990), the traumatic experience is overwhelming and can occur either as a single catastrophic event or as a
series of ordeals.

Ehrlich et al. (1980) define trauma as an emotional shock, produc-
ing a lasting effect upon a person. Monahon (1993) compares this
traumatic effect to a childhood wound: "The wound is often invisible,
internal; no X rays define the damage" (p. 7).

Psychological trauma has been defined by the American Psychiatric Association (APA) in the *Diagnostic and Statistical Manual of*

Mental Disorders, Third Edition, Revis
as an occurrence which is outside the sc
rience and which would be notably distr
DSM-IV (APA, 1994) provides further
by requiring that the individual has unde
faced with an event that has been threat
someone else. In addition, it prescribes
must consist of intense fear, helplessne

Social trauma is a term sometimes us
a historic process can leave an entire
Baró, 1989), as in the case of long-term
individualized accounts of trauma are cc
understanding traumatized cultures (Jer

We may not always agree on the "cor
but one thing is for certain: we know it v
frightening image of a tornado and the
houses. It could be the sound of infants
rages out of control, or the onslaught of
It could be a rash of gunfire and the sigl
ground. It could also be the ongoing expe
manization as a result of such acts as pol
violence.

If these horrible experiences and the
pany them are too much for adults to stc
children must often endure in this turbu

Traumatic incidents can strike any re
vary in size, complexity, and scope, but t
trous, and their effects can be devastating
that can last a lifetime.

THREATS OR ACTS OI

On September 11, 2001, as parents,
pared for a new school year, a sequence
America. President George W. Bush firs
was reading to children in a classroom. I
the world would never forget:

- American Airlines Flight 11 from Boston crashed into the North Tower of the World Trade Center in New York. Eighty-one passengers and eleven crew tragically lost their lives. Those who worked for companies located in the crash zone of the tower were killed on impact. Many individuals on the upper floors had no chance of survival due to unrelenting fires that cut off escape routes.
- United Airlines Flight 175 crashed into the South Tower of the World Trade Center causing a devastating explosion. Fifty-six passengers and nine crew aboard the flight perished. It became evident that the dual catastrophes were not accidental.
- An estimated 3,019 civilians lost their lives.
- In responding to the disaster, 347 firefighters and 71 law enforcement officers were killed in the line of duty.
- American Airlines Flight 77 from Washington, DC, to Los Angeles crashed into the Pentagon. A portion of the Pentagon collapsed. Fifty-eight passengers, six crew members, and 125 Pentagon employees were added to the devastation and loss of life.
- United Airlines Flight 93 crashed eighty miles southeast of Pittsburgh, killing all forty-five people on board. Speculation suggests that its intended target may have been the White House.

Life in New York City fell into turmoil as the Twin Towers collapsed, releasing clouds of debris and smoke. Reports told of bodies strewn on the pavement and blood splattered everywhere. Waves of panic crossed the nation as teachers grappled to find the right words to reassure students and to quiet their fears. Parents who were nowhere near the area of the devastation felt the need to leave work early or stop whatever they were doing to be closer to their children and protect them.

Terrorism

> No other form of violence approaches the mystery and uniqueness of terrorism. For the relatively simple act of hijacking a plane, or kidnapping a person, or blowing up a building, a whole sequence of global events can unfold that can last months, years, or even decades beyond that brief moment of violence. (Simon, 2001, p. 5)

The four planes that crashed on Sept
States were hijacked as part of a terror
people from approximately eighty nat
Antigua to Zimbabwe—were killed in
sands of children were orphaned.

The threat of terrorism continues to I
the United States but the internationa
2003, 190 international terrorist attacl
from the 198 attacks that occurred in 2
from the 346 attacks that occurred in 20
2004). Also in 2003, 307 people lost tl
1,593 people were wounded, down fr
2,013 wounded during 2002, as well as
people dead and 2,283 wounded (U.S
Thousands of the fatalities recorded for
11 attacks on New York, Washington,

For the victims of violence, war an
able. A blast in a marketplace could j
bomb as an artillery shell (Silver and I
City bombing, for instance, killed twe
Americans killed in combat during the
(Michel and Herbeck, 2001).

Acts of War and Armed Conflict

> For most of us, the experience of
> by comforting euphemisms. Our
> by images associated with words l
> bravery, casualties, national securi
> and defeat. As those who have be
> real essence of real war is terro:
> ment, peeing in your pants from I
> guts of your friends, chaos so pro
> recognize it for what it is. (Garba
> 1991, p. 7)

Wars were once fought between ar:
more children than soldiers have bee
armed conflict. During that period, an
were killed in armed conflicts, between

BOX 1.1.
Examples of Actual Incidents of Terrorism

- May 2004: Four young Israeli children and their pregnant mother were killed in a terrorist attack in Gaza.
- April 2004: In Baghdad, Iraq, suicide attacks resulted in the deaths of at least sixty-eight people, including as many as twenty-three children who were on their way to school.
- March 2004: Terrorists exploded ten bombs on four trains at different locations in Madrid, Spain. Passengers consisted of students and school children; 191 people were killed and more than 2,000 were wounded.
- March 2003: Seventeen people were killed, including one child and eight teenagers, by a suicide bombing on a bus in Haifa en route to Haifa University; 53 people were injured in the attack.
- November 2002: Eleven people were killed and fifty were injured in Jerusalem when a suicide bomber exploded on a bus filled with passengers, including school children.
- October 2002: A car bomb exploded outside a discotheque in Bali, Indonesia, killing at least 202 people and injuring 300 more.
- August 2002: In Pakistan, gunmen attacked a Christian school that was being attended by children of missionaries from various parts of the world. Six people were killed and one was injured.
- June 2002: A bus transporting several children to school in Jerusalem became the target of a suicide bomber. Nineteen people were killed and more than fifty people were injured during the explosion.
- March 2002: Twenty-five people were injured when a suicide bomber exploded near a bus in Jerusalem. Many of the passengers were high school students.
- February 2002: Four people, including two teenagers, were killed and twenty-seven were injured in a suicide bomb attack on a pizzeria in Karnei Shomron in the West Bank.
- October 2001: Six gunmen attacked a church in Bahawalpur, Pakistan, killing fifteen Pakistani Christians.
- August 2001: A suicide bombing at a pizzeria in Jerusalem claimed the lives of fifteen people, including seven children, and injured 130 others.
- May 2001: Two teenagers were stoned to death in Wadi Haritun cave near Teqoa (Israeli settlement) in the West Bank. A terrorist group claimed responsibility.

(continued)

(continued)

- December 2000: In India, a grenac
  rity vehicle missed its target and ex
  Pattan, injuring twelve persons, ac
- October 2000: Seventeen U.S. sai
  attack against the destroyer USS
  Aden; thirty-nine others were injure
- July 2000: In Germany, unidentifi
  refuge shelter housing Albanian K
  dren.
- January 2000: In Namibia, unident
  vehicles in Rundu, killing three chil
  ents.
- August 1998: At least 291 people l
  of the U.S. embassy in Kenya, wh
  people. Ten others were killed anc
  second U.S. embassy bombing in
- April 1995: A truck bomb destroyed
  Building in Oklahoma City, killing
  others. Nineteen children, ages fi
  building collapse. Many of the child
  on the second floor at the time of
  were carried out of the building ar
  side, covered with blankets. Their p
  use as a temporary morgue" (Miche
  A total of 219 children lost a parent
  phaned.
- February 1993: The World Trade C
  badly damaged when a car bomb pl
  nated in an underground garage,
  1,000 injured.

The possibility of a terrorist attack i
destruction (WMD)—chemical, biolc
(CBRN)— also remains real.

(continued)

In October 2003, a metallic container was found at a South Carolina postal facility with the biological agent ricin in it. The container was placed inside an envelope along with a threatening note.

In January 2003, six Algerians were arrested in London for attempting to develop or manufacture a chemical weapon. Following the arrests, authorities discovered traces of ricin in their apartment.

In June 2002, a man was arrested for possession of ricin in his Spokane Valley office cubicle. His co-workers notified FBI officials after discovering documents on "how to kill," undetectable poisons, and bomb making that had been printed out from his computer. Further investigation of his office produced test tubes, glass jars, castor beans, and approximately 1 gram of ricin.

- Since October 2001, a series of bioterrorism incidents using *Bacillus anthracis* spores sent through the mail resulted in at least twenty-two anthrax cases and five deaths.
- In 1995, the release of nerve agent sarin in a crowded subway station in the center of Tokyo, Japan, convinced the world to pay heed to the reality of chemical or biological weapons use on a civilian population. The intentional use of this nerve gas in this incident resulted in twelve deaths and the injury of 5,700 children and adults.
- In 1995, the Federal Bureau of Investigation uncovered a terrorist effort to release a chlorine gas bomb in the Disneyland theme park in California.

physically disabled, more than 5 million became refugees, and more than 12 million were uprooted from their homes (United Nations Children's Fund [UNICEF], 1995).

In times of conflict, anything that can be done to adults, no matter how monstrous, can also be visited on children. Children have been tortured as a way of punishing their parents—or sometimes just for entertainment (UNICEF, 1996). In many parts of the world children have been recruited as soldiers, given drugs and weapons, and desensitized to the pain of others. Their opportunity to be raised in a society that nurtures and promotes their development has been stolen from them.

War violates every right of a child—
with family and community, the right to
opment of personality, and the right
(Machel, 1996). Generations of childr
ously injured, both physically and emo
conflict. Countless others die as a resu
exacerbated by the disruption of health

A great number of conflicts occur in
nations where children are already vuln
cieties—homes, health facilities, and e
tutions—is ripped apart all in the name

BOX 1.2.
Examples of Actual Inc
and Armed Co

- December 2003: Six children in A
  bombing raid between the U.S. mili
- March 2003: The United States–led
  tion. Many of the military casualtie
  whose children were left fatherless
  Iraqi soldiers and civilians killed c
  mated to be higher than in the 19
  Several children were included amc
- March 2003: A twelve-year-old Iraq
  his parents, his brother, and seven
  coalition bombing raid near Baghda
- July 2002: American forces were res
  least forty-eight civilians when a str
  Afghanistan. Twenty-five of the dea
  attending a wedding.
- April 2002: Israeli forces launched n
  ian refuge camp in Jenin resulting in
  100 people, including both Palestin
  However, some reports stated that
  tims were women and children.
- Continued conflict in Afghanistan
  deaths and injuries, as well as mass

(continued)

and prolonged drought. More than 10 million children have suffered due to the civil war and political instability that has existed in Afghanistan for twenty-three years. Millions of land mines and unexploded ordnances remain throughout the country and have killed or wounded an estimated 400,000 Afghans. Thirty-four percent of these casualties involve children.

- 2001: An eleven-year-old Palestinian boy was shot to death during a clash between Palestinian and Israeli forces.
- 2001: Two Israeli teenagers were killed by a suicide bomber as they waited for a bus to take them to seminary school.
- November 2001: Five Palestinian children were killed when they encountered unexploded ordnance on their way to school in Gaza.
- August 2000: In Bogota, Colombia, at least six children between the ages of five and fifteen were killed when they were caught in crossfire between Colombian government forces and a rebel group. Three other students and a teacher were wounded.
- 1998: Countless ethnic Albanians were killed during the war in Kosovo. Men were executed by the Serb military; families were forced to witness unspeakable atrocities; and massive numbers of refugees, many of whom were women and children, were forced from their homes. Upon their return home, several children were maimed by land mines and unexploded ordnances that were left behind by Serbian soldiers.

Gender-Based Violence

Girls are continually at risk of sexual assault during armed conflict. Boys are also affected. Gender-based violence is often used as a tactic of war to cause mass fear and to coerce civilians into fleeing from their homes. Other forms of gender-based violence include prostitution, mutilation, trafficking, domestic violence, and ethnic cleansing through impregnation. Some children have even been forced to witness the sexual assault of their parents.

In Bosnia, Herzegovina, and Croatia, it has been a deliberate policy to rape adolescent girls and to coerce them into giving birth to the enemy's child. In Rwanda, rape has been systematically used as a weapon of ethnic cleansing to destroy community ties (UNICEF, 1996).

Girls who have been impregnated as ;
cized by their families and communit
other choice but to give up their babies

Homicide

> Millions of children struggle to s
> conditions on the streets of the w
> geles to Sao Paulo to Manila. Gun;
> ing parts of daily life. (UNICEF, 1

Exacerbated by the ready availability
lence has become a public health issue
children everywhere are feeling its ver
States, consider the child who is forced t
mother, or the teenager whose brother is
yard. In Guatemala City, consider the "s
by a police officer, or, in Sri Lanka, the
his mother during armed conflict. Violer
children in all corners of the world.

An international comparative analys
International Collaborative Effort (ICE
Centers for Disease Control and Preven
lowing findings:

- The death rate from firearm injuries
  teen per 100,000, was more than tv
  son countries (Australia, Canada, D
  France, Israel, New Zealand, the
  Scotland).
- In four of the comparison countries
  Israel, and France) firearms were th
  jury death from ages fifteen to twe
- In all the countries except the Unit
  were primarily (51 to 93 percent) s
- In the United States, the majority o
  homicides (62 percent).
- The homicide rate in the United Sta
  four to nine times the rates in comp

of homicides in the United States were committed with fire-arms.

- In the United States, the firearm injury death rate, twenty-seven per 100,000, was four to six times the rates in Norway, Israel, and France.
- The Netherlands, England, Wales, and Scotland had notably low death rates by firearms, with less than one death per 100,000 people.
- New Zealand had a low overall rate of firearm-related deaths.
- Unintentional injury accounted for 61 to 72 percent, suicide for 21 to 31 percent, and homicide for 1 to 6 percent of injury deaths in all countries—except in the United States, where homicide accounted for 15 percent of the deaths. (Fingerhut et al., 1998)

In the United States, homicide is the second leading cause of death among fifteen- to twenty-four-year-olds, the fifth leading cause of death among ten- to fourteen-year-olds, and the fourth leading cause of death among one- to nine-year-olds (National Center for Injury Prevention and Control [NCIPC], n.d.). In most murders of a young child, a family member killed the child, while in most murders of an older child (ages fifteen to seventeen), the perpetrator was an acquaintance of the victim or was unknown to law enforcement authorities (U.S. Department of Justice [DOJ], Bureau of Justice Statistics, 1996).

The number of homicides of children under age five increased between 1976 and 2000 but has been on the decline recently. Most of the children killed are male, and most of the offenders are male (Fox and Zawitz, 1998). The number of children under the age of five murdered from 1976 to 2000 (Fox and Zawitz, 1998) include

- 30 percent who were killed by mothers,
- 31 percent who were killed by fathers,
- 7 percent who were killed by other relatives,
- 23 percent who were killed by male acquaintances, and
- 3 percent who were killed by strangers.

Twelve percent were killed by perpetrators whose relationship to them was unknown.

We live in violent times. Violence
race, ethnicity, sex, class, or geographic
immune to its disastrous effects. Vio
homes, their communities, and their fa
there, violence will come knocking at

Since the late 1990s, schools in the
dated by violent incidents. Increasing
weapons to settle conflicts, which all
presence of metal detectors, the patrol o
schools are woeful indicators of this fac
have escalated dramatically and are jus
suburban communities as they are in th

BOX 1.3.
Examples of Actual Incident

- April 2004: In Pennsylvania, an eig
  reportedly hanged himself in a high
  of ninth-grade students discovered
- March 2004: In Washington, a thi
  shot and killed himself in a scho
  twenty other students were in atter
- March 2004: In Nebraska, a teen
  tempted murder after police found
  twenty homemade bombs, a rifle,
  wanted to harm everyone at his hig
  of three of his friends.
- February 2004: In Pennsylvania, 1C
  val gangs as children were on t
  school. A ten-year-old student was
  crossing guard was injured.
- April 2003: A fourteen-year-old boy
  fore taking his own life.
- October 2002: A series of sniper at
  ington, DC, area. The youngest vic
  boy who was shot and critically wou
- April 2002: An expelled student sh
  ers, two other students, a police off
  in eastern Germany.

(continued)

- 2001: An eighteen-year-old senior wounded three students and two teachers in a shooting at an El Cajon, California, high school.
- March 2001: A fifteen-year-old student killed two students and injured thirteen others at a high school in Santee, California.
- February 2001: A man attacked three women and five children with a machete at an elementary school in York, Pennsylvania.
- 2000: A thirteen-year-old student shot and killed a teacher at a middle school in Lake Worth, Florida.
- March 2000: A student killed a teacher and shot himself at a boarding school in southern Germany.
- February 2000: A six-year-old child fatally shot another six-year-old child at an elementary school in Flint, Michigan.
- 1999: A fourteen-year-old Canadian boy shot and killed a seventeen-year-old student and injured another student in a high school in Canada.
- 1999: A student killed two people and wounded nine others at an elementary school playground in San Diego, California.
- July 1999: Three teachers were killed at a school in Johannesburg, South Africa.
- May 1999: A fifteen-year-old student shot and wounded six of his classmates at his high school in Conyers, Georgia.
- April 1999: In Littleton, Colorado, two students packed with guns and explosives murdered twelve students and a teacher and injured at least twenty-three others before taking their own lives.
- May 1998: In Springfield, Oregon, a fifteen-year-old boy killed two students and wounded twenty-two others at his high school.
- March 1998: Two boys in Jonesboro, Arkansas, armed with several weapons, fatally shot four students and a teacher. Ten others were injured.
- December 1997: In Paducah, Kentucky, a fifteen-year-old boy killed three students and injured five others.
- October 1997: In Mississippi, a seventeen-year-old boy killed two students and injured others.
- March 1997: Hundreds of students at two schools in Yemen were shot by a man carrying an assault weapon. Eight people were killed, including six children.
- February 1997: In Bethel, Alaska, a sixteen-year-old boy, with the help of two friends, murdered a student and the principal at the high school, which they attended. Two other students were injured.
- March 1996: A man killed sixteen children, a teacher, and himself at a primary school in Scotland.

The National Center for Education
ported the following data on crime in

- 2001-2002: Seventeen school-a
  school-associated violent death.
- 2001: Eight percent of students ag
  ported that they had been bullied a
  up from 5 percent in 1999.
- 2001: Students ages twelve to ei
  764,000 violent crimes at school
  and aggravated and simple assault
  olent crimes (rape, sexual assaul
  sault). Away from school, students
  violent crimes, including 290,000
- Between July 1, 1999, and June
  associated violent deaths occurre
  ing twenty-four homicides, sixte
  aged children. Six of these violen
- For the period July 1, 1992, to Jun
  ated violent deaths occurred on t
  tary or secondary schools. Of th
  homicides and 43 were suicides o
  to nineteen).
- Away from school, a total of 1,92
  to nineteen were committed durir

The percentage of adolescents inv
mains high. Every individual, family, a
violent acts and juvenile crimes that exi
many children have become so overwh
concentrate in the classroom and belie
ons to school to protect themselves.

Suicide

The rise in suicide among the worlc
and a reflection of the many ills that pla
employment, drug abuse, breakdown
spread hunger, and armed conflict. In th

ropean countries, youth suicide has become a major public health concern.

Young people who see no alternative to their negative plights will set out to eradicate their lives by any means necessary, which includes shooting themselves with firearms as noted in the United States and Norway, and poisoning themselves as noted in England, Wales, Scotland, New Zealand, Australia, and Sri Lanka. Other means of suicide have included suffocation, as noted in the Netherlands, France, Israel, and Canada; jumping from extreme heights, as noted in Hong Kong and Singapore; and plunging into the Han River in South Korea.

BOX 1.4. Recent Suicide Statistics

- Suicide rates have varied immensely from a high in Hungary and Sri Lanka to a low in Egypt and Kuwait (Lester, 1997).
- In Sri Lanka, deaths are common among youths who are often exposed to those who have previously attempted to take their own lives (Eddleston, Rezvi, and Hawton, 1998).
- In Ireland, suicide among young people ages fifteen to twenty-four competes with cancer as the leading cause of death (Birchard, 1998).
- Every week ten young Australians are reported to commit suicide, and 1,000 attempt to do so (Loff and Cordner, 1998).
- During 1998, suicides were expected to exceed the number of deaths from traffic accidents in South Korea (Watts, 1998).

In the United States, suicide is the third leading cause of death among fifteen- to twenty-four-year-olds, as well as among ten- to fourteen-year-olds (NCIPC, n.d.). For every young person who actually commits suicide, many more give it serious consideration or make some type of attempt, which places them at risk for the likelihood of completed suicides in the future.

Being exposed to an environment in which your friends or acquaintances have thought of attempting suicide—and at least one person may have already done so—impacts the lives of all young people. Many young people who attempt suicide do not wish to die. Their attempts are a frantic plea for attention and a cry for help. Due to rash behavior and miscalculation, they often die before anyone can reach out to them.

Child Abuse

The Child Abuse Prevention and Tre
child abuse and neglect as, at a minimu
act resulting in imminent risk of serious
or emotional harm, sexual abuse, or ex;
under the age of eighteen, unless the ch
in which the child resides specifies a ¡
volving sexual abuse) by a parent or
ployee of a residential facility or any s
home care) who is responsible for t
Clearing House on Child Abuse and N

> Most parents try to do the best th
> some cannot, or will not meet thei
> Neglected children starve becau:
> them; they freeze when they are l
> temperatures; and, left alone, the}
> neglected children fail to grow pr
> tively abused. They are kicked, b
> walls and radiators, strangled, su
> even buried alive. They are hum
> people who are supposed to nurt
> 1993, p. 283)

The U.S. Department of Health and F
ministration for Children and Families (
reau (CB) (n.d.) reported the following
glect:

- Nationally, an estimated 896,000 c
  and neglect in 2002. Of these, mo
  suffered neglect, nearly 20 percen
  10 percent were sexually abused;
  were associated with additional ty
- Children in the age group of birth
  victimization rate at 16.0 victims ¡
- A nationally estimated 1,400 child;
  2002—a rate of two children per 1(

tion, and 76 percent of these fatalities were among children younger than four years of age.

Commercial Sexual Exploitation

Commercial sexual exploitation is the exploitation, for sexual purposes and for financial or in-kind profit, of children (defined in the United Nations Convention on the Rights of the Child as a person under the age of eighteen, or as otherwise defined by an individual country).

Commercial sexual exploitation of children is an extremely hazardous form of child labor, an abuse of power over children, and a way to dominate them (World Congress Against the Commercial Sexual Exploitation of Children, n.d.). A growing number of children around the world are subjected to sexual exploitation and sexual abuse daily. Children are treated as both sexual and commercial objects. The commercial sexual exploitation of children constitutes a form of coercion and violence against children and amounts to forced labor and contemporary forms of slavery (World Congress Against the Commercial Sexual Exploitation of Children, n.d.).

The exact nature of exploitation varies from one nation to another. The World Congress Against the Commercial Sexual Exploitation of Children (n.d.) provides the following descriptions which indicate the type of exploitation most generally recognized as predominating in each region:

- In Asia, local men sexually exploit children for profit by using them as prostitutes or involving them in "sex tourism"—men traveling to other countries in order to have sexual relations with children. Occasionally, family members or friends sell children into the sex trade under the mistaken belief that the children are going to be employed as domestic servants and earn money for the family. Sometimes kidnapping and trafficking of children occur across borders or from rural to urban areas. The children are moved around from one location to another in order to effectively "disappear" from sight.
- In South America, children who believe they have no choice but to earn employment on the streets may, eventually, choose or be forced into the sex trade. They become prey to pimps and others

who are seeking to sexually exploit
are told that they will be afforded pro
just a cover-up for abuse, violence, a

• In Europe, children are trafficked ac
  Europe from poorer countries in the
  where more of a market exists.

• In Africa, it has been reported that cl
  vants are often sexually exploited. (
  restaurants, and brothels have experi-

• In the Middle East, children are often
  under the guise of becoming employe
  dren are also given into early marria:
  tivities. An exchange of money or cor
  in such situations.

• In addition, reports suggest that chil
  being sexually exploited for commerc
  and by men in surrounding communi

According to UNICEF's State of th
least 100,000 children in the United S
have been involved in child prostitution

SCHOOL BUS ACC

Millions of children begin and end th
the school bus. Some make it safely to
not. In the United States, school bus oc
fatalities than those occupying other n
the sudden, unexpected death of a chilc
still a tragedy.

Since 1991, 1,479 people have died in
crashes—an average of 134 fatalities p
who lost their lives in those crashes (68
other vehicles involved (National High
tration [NHTSA], Department of Trans
occupants (pedestrians, bicyclists, etc.)
the deaths, and occupants of school trans
for 9 percent (NHTSA, DOT, n.d.).

Since 1991, 210 school-age pedestrians (younger than nineteen years old) have died in school-transportation-related crashes. Nearly two-thirds (64 percent) were killed by school buses, 5 percent by vehicles functioning as school buses, and 30 percent by other vehicles involved in the crashes. One-half (50 percent) of all school-age pedestrians killed in school bus–related crashes were between the ages of five and seven (NHTSA, DOT, n.d.).

BOX 1.5.
Examples of Actual School Bus-Related Incidents

- April 2004: In Turkey, at least eighteen people were killed, including seven school children, when a train slammed into their school bus at a railway crossing.
- April 2004: In Colombia, a fifty-ton excavator fell from a slope onto a school bus, killing one adult and twenty-two children who were on their way home from school.
- April 2004: In France, two teenagers from a North Carolina Youth Soccer Association lost their lives when their tour bus ran into a ditch and overturned.
- December 2003: In southwest China, a bus loaded with elementary and middle school children plunged off a mountain road into a river, killing at least seventeen people.
- October 2003: In Indonesia, at least fifty-four people lost their lives when their bus caught on fire after colliding with a truck and a minivan. Most of the victims were children.
- October 2002: A bus carrying a high school football team crashed in Kansas, killing an assistant coach and injuring several students and adults.
- August 2002: In Nigeria, at least sixteen people were killed when their bus crashed. Fifteen of the victims were children.
- 2001: Two students were killed and nine other people were injured when an eighteen-wheeler crashed into their school bus in Arkansas.
- 2000: A school bus crash in Malaysia left fifteen people dead; thirteen of them were children.
- 2000: A school bus was hit by a train along the Tennessee–Georgia border, killing three children and injuring five others.
- 2000: A snowplow struck a school bus in Wyoming, killing two children and injuring three others.

(continued)

(continued)

- 1999: At least eleven students an
  school bus accident in Kenya.
- 1999: Eleven students were injure
  exploded on their school bus.
- 1999: A bus in Austria with Hungari
  whom were teenagers, was invo
  eighteen passengers dead and thir
- December 1998: A van loaded with
  state of Georgia, collided with a truc
  a stop sign. One preschooler was k
  were injured.
- April 1998: A school bus was invc
  other vehicles during a rainy day ir
  children were killed as a result.
- March 1998: Ten students in India w
  between their bus, which had blov
  driving the opposite way. Twenty-c
  also killed.

FIRE INCIDI

Imagine the sound of crackling flame
a fireplace or the smell of chestnuts roa
ine the taste of sweet, sticky marshn
toasted in a campfire or the warm sens;
a bonfire on a cold, winter day. These
some of the more memorable and enjo

Unfortunately, dark images of fire
well—images which are, probably, best
a neighborhood church after it has burn
flesh of the victim of a hate crime. Ima;
a household being engulfed by flames,
rious hands of a child, or the smell of a;
ruins of the place you once called hom

The United States has one of the hig
dustrialized world at 12 deaths per 1
States Fire Administration [USFA],
ment Agency [FEMA] "The Overall Fi

are killed each year by fire than floods, hurricanes, earthquakes, and all other natural disasters combined. Between 1992 and 2001, exclusive of the events of September 11, an average of 4,266 Americans lost their lives and another 24,913 were injured annually due to fire (USFA, FEMA, "Facts on Fire," n.d.).

BOX 1.6.
Examples of Actual Fire-Related Incidents

- July 2004: In Southern India, at least eighty children lost their lives in a school fire and more than a hundred were wounded.
- April 2003: In Russia, a fire claimed the lives of at least thirty children at a boarding school.
- In 2003, a fire erupted at a nightclub in Rhode Island, United States, killing 98 people and injuring more than 180. Adolescents were included among the casualties.
- 2003: A fire killed twenty-eight hearing-impaired children at a Russian boarding school while many of them were sleeping. Twenty-nine other children were injured.
- 2003: At least twenty-one students, ages eleven through eighteen, and one teacher were killed when a fire consumed their school in Russia. Ten other children sustained injuries while trying to leap from the windows.
- 2002: A fire, which was started in a marketplace near an army munitions dump in Lagos, Nigeria, resulted in massive explosions. More than 1,100 people were killed while trying to escape. Many of the fatalities were children and infants.
- March 2001: In Kenya, at least fifty-eight children burned to death due to a suspected arson attack on their school.
- 1999: Twenty-three kindergarten children were killed and two other children and a teacher were injured in a fire near Seoul, Korea.
- 1998: A fire erupted at a Halloween party for high school students in Sweden. Sixty-two people, mostly adolescents, lost their lives.
- 1998: Twenty-three children and five adults were killed in a fire at an orphanage in the Philippines.
- 1996: One hundred forty-nine youth, mostly college students, perished in a fire at a disco in the Philippines. They were celebrating the end of the school year.

Children set over 100,000 fires each
the fires that kill children are set by chil
under the age of five are curious about
as a natural exploration of the unknow
FEMA, "Curious Kids," n.d.).

NATURAL DIS

At this very moment, somewhen
shaking violently. In other places,
a froth and permeating the air w
storms wipe out roads, bridges an
lages, causing havoc and destru
contrast, there are places on other
ing seems to be moving. Life itsel
lyzed by the dead hand of droug
embracing curfew. (World Meteor
United Nations, "WMO: For a Sa

Natural disasters can happen sudder
of their own. Wildfires can rage out of
age to forestry; tornadoes can touch de
their path; hurricanes can leave trails o
ther deaths and homelessness; and seve
causing damage to lives, crops, and ho
Among the different types of natu
storms, droughts, and earthquakes are 1
by landslides and storms. Several millio
lessness, disaster-induced ill health, sev
sonal tragedies in the wake of natural
left shaking their heads in disbelief, wo
could occur in just a blink of an eye.
Every region of the world is prone to
and no culture is immune to the expe
present themselves in the aftermath.
year, and children are often among the

BOX 1.7.
Examples of Actual Natural Disasters
and Levels of Impact

Events during 2004

• Flash floods in Texas killed six people, including two toddlers, after a wave of thunderstorms swept across North Texas.
• At least 198 people were killed when cyclone Gafilo hit northern Madagascar.

Events during 2003

• Parts of central United States, extending from Kansas eastward to Tennessee, were inundated by fierce storms, flash floods, and tornadoes. At least forty-four people lost their lives as a result.
• Approximately 167 people were killed in an earthquake that struck Turkey. Eighty-four children, all boys (ages twelve to eighteen), and one teacher were among the victims when their boarding school collapsed on top of their sleeping bodies.
• An avalanche in British Columbia took the lives of seven adolescents.
• An estimated 43,200 people were killed and 30,000 injured in an earthquake that struck southeastern Iran. This was believed to be the largest earthquake to occur in this area in more than 2,000 years.
• In the Democratic Republic of Congo, lightning struck a school, killing eleven students and injuring seventy-three.

Events during 2002

• An earthquake struck southern Italy, resulting in the deaths of twenty-six children and one teacher at an elementary school. The children were in their first-grade classroom preparing for a Halloween party when their ceiling collapsed.
• An earthquake hit Afghanistan, killing approximately 1,800 people and injuring nearly 4,000.
• At least 1,000 people lost their lives during a heat wave in central and southeastern India.

(continued)

(continued)

- At least forty-five people were kille
  the eastern part of Democratic Rep
- Severe weather and tornadoes occ
  and Ohio Valley region in the Unite
  thirty-six deaths.
- In Bangladesh, up to 300 people dr
  in a storm. It was one of the wor
  1980s.

Events during 2001

- A flood in Algeria left at least 579 p
- Over 400 people were injured in the
  States) when an earthquake struc
  center.
- A major earthquake in northweste
  confirmed dead.
- An earthquake occurred off the co
  least 844 people lost their lives and
  vador.
- An earthquake near the coast of P
  killed and 1,368 injured.
- Hurricane Allison was responsible
  related deaths in the United States
  died in Texas, one in Louisiana, on
  Florida.
- Severe drought conditions and flash
  deaths of at least 500 people and l

Events during 2000

- Approximately 103 people were kil
  during an earthquake in Indonesia.
- Hurricane Gordon killed at least tw
  mala.
- In Alabama, at least five tornadoes
  seventy-five, and destroyed hundre

(continued)

Events during 1999

- A major earthquake struck Turkey, resulting in over 15,000 deaths.
- At least 2,101 people lost their lives due to a massive earthquake that struck Taiwan.
- Flooding in North Carolina caused by Hurricane Floyd claimed the lives of at least forty-eight people.
- Severe drought affected the United States, portions of Russia, the Middle East, Ivory Coast, Uganda, and Spain.
- Significant tornado outbreaks in the United States and South Africa resulted in several fatalities.
- Landslides claimed the lives of people in Indonesia, Pakistan, and the Philippines.
- Many deaths occurred and homes were destroyed due to flooding in Brazil, Colombia, China, the Philippines, the Ukraine, India, and Iran.
- Forest fires in India and China claimed a number of lives.
- At least 400 people died in Pakistan due to a cyclone.
- Approximately 150 people in the United States and 140 people in India lost their lives in heat waves.

Events during 1998

Numerous extreme climatic events occurred in 1998. Powerful hurricanes, tornadoes, wildfires, and floods occurred throughout the world, leaving massive devastation behind. This devastation resulted in thousands of fatalities, homelessness, agricultural losses, and a massive outbreak of disease across the globe. Economic costs amounted to billions of (U.S.) dollars.

- February 1998: A series of tornadoes swept across central Florida. Forty-two deaths occurred and over 800 residences were destroyed.
- March 1998: A tornado touched down in Georgia, damaging two schools and numerous homes and buildings. At least thirteen people were killed.

(continued)

(continued)

- April 1998: Severe weather struck ir
  sissippi River Valley, bringing heavy
  at least eleven people and injured
  heavily affected states included Tenr
  Alabama, and Illinois.
- The United States had seven landfa
  canes Bonnie, Earl, Georges, France
  Charley and Hermine. There were !
  and 30 percent more tropical storm
  anic and Atmospheric Administratio
- Hurricane Mitch (category 5) was t
  cane on record for the Atlantic ba
  death and destruction for portions c
  least 11,000 people and leaving mc
  ther homeless or severely affected (
  ter [NCDC], NOAA, "Mitch," n.d.).
- Hurricane Georges was the second
  gest hurricane within the Atlantic ba
  Its seventeen-day journey resulted i
  from the northeast Caribbean regior
  and an estimated 602 fatalities main
  lic and Haiti (National Hurricane Ce
- During February, California was stru
  estimated seventeen storm-related
  the winter and thirty-five counties we
  areas (NOAA, NCDC, n.d.).
- Southern Texas was struck by tropic
  with flooding rains, resulting in at le
  and Mexico (NCDC, NOAA, 1999).
- China suffered massive flooding dur
  ple were killed by the floods—the sec
  in more than 130 years. The floods l
  less, caused $20 billion (U.S.) in es
  fected 240 million people (NCDC, N
  n.d.).
- For 1998, a total of 21,688 earthquak
  8,928 deaths were estimated (Unite
  [USGS], National Earthquake Inforn

OTHER TRAUMAS FACED BY CHILDREN

Several other kinds of traumatic incidents affect children but go beyond the scope of this book and, therefore, will not be discussed in detail. They include the following:

- Female genital mutilation through the process of circumcision, excision, and infibulation occurs as a means of ensuring cleanliness and fidelity. This practice has negative, lifelong consequences to the physical and psychological health of girls and women, and is sometimes deadly. Female genital mutilation continues to be practiced in much of Sub-Saharan Africa, in varying degrees in Egypt, Oman, Yemen, and a few other countries in the Middle East.
- Abuses against street children (as young as five years old) are committed throughout the world.
- Child labor abuses and slavery are widespread. Countless numbers of children worldwide (as young as five years old) are forced to work at often illegal, hazardous, and exploitative jobs. The majority of these child laborers live in Asia, Africa, and Latin America. There have also been incidents of children in Sudan being abducted during armed conflicts and forced to become domestic slaves.

SUMMARY

1. According to Terr (1990), the traumatic experience is overwhelming and can occur either as a single catastrophic event or as a series of ordeals.
2. *Social trauma* is a term used to define the way in which a historic process can leave an entire population affected (Martín-Baró, 1989), as in the case of long-term civil warfare.
3. Among the different types of natural disasters, floods, tropical storms, droughts, and earthquakes are the most destructive, followed by landslides and storms.
4. Each year, fire kills more Americans than floods, hurricanes, earthquakes, and all natural disasters combined.

5. From 1988 to 1998, half of all sch
   school bus–related crashes were b
   seven (NHTSA, DOT, n.d.).
6. The death rate from firearm injuries ▪
   per 100,000 was more than twice the
   tries (Australia, Canada, Denmark, F
   rael, New Zealand, the Netherlands,
   National Center for Health Statistic:
7. In the United States and many Euro
   has become a major public health co
8. The commercial sexual exploitation
   of coercion and violence against ch
   labor and contemporary forms of sla·
   the Commercial Sexual Exploitatior
9. Wars were once fought between arn
   1980s far more children than soldi·
   abled (UNICEF, 1995).

Chapter 2

Developmental Considerations

I thought to myself that the scream of the newborn had something of a question in it. It was like a signal sent out by the newcomer to see if he had arrived at the right place. The sound most similar to a newborn's scream is the sound of children, which is why children in my village are required to cry out in confirmation of the newborn's arrival. This confirmation satisfies something in the psyche of the newborn, who is now ready to surrender to being present in this world. I have often wondered, what would happen to the newborn if there were no answer? Can infants recover from the damage done to their souls as a result of a message at birth that they are on their own? (Somé, 1998, p. 93)

Worldwide, children from infancy through adolescence are susceptible to traumatic experiences of varying degrees. In attempting to understand the impact of these experiences on children and how to respond appropriately, developmental factors must be taken into account.

PSYCHOSOCIAL STAGES OF EGO DEVELOPMENT

Trust versus Mistrust (Birth to Age Three)

An infant's early experiences are critical and must be handled with the utmost care. It is during this stage that the infant learns to develop a sense of basic trust—the willingness to let his or her mother out of sight without undue anxiety or rage, because she has become an inner certainty and an outer predictability (Erikson, 1950).

The infant, having been fed and nur███
accustomed to routine and a sense of
confident to test out other people and o██
infant eventually comes to the realizat
familiar adults and that the world is re██

Not so for the traumatized infant, hc
cannot rely on a mother who is in flig
nourished herself to provide the nurtu
needs. These children cannot rely on a ███
he attempts to take his own life. They
feels she must abandon them because t
rapist who impregnated her, or beca██
brought her a sense of shame, loss of
What then is the fate of the traumatize

Violence against the mother was not█
rience among children following the
Iraqi Kurdistan (Ahmad et al., 2000). A
a trauma is frequent or severe enougl
thrive; it may also result in many relate

Scheeringa and Zeanah (1995) repoi
traumatic stress disorder was present i
dlers when traumas involved threats t█
traumas produced more fears, displa█
arousal symptoms than traumas that d
givers.

If an infant's attachment to a parent ɕ
paired by a traumatic incident, serious
can arise. According to Erikson (1950)
an overwhelming sense of basic mistr█
infant's cries are no longer responded t
ticipate being nurtured and comforted; ɐ
stability and routine are no longer exist
world is unpredictable and others are nc

Kiser et al. (1988) conducted a stud
years who allegedly had been sexually
trust of people was evident in these cl
difficulties with personal social relatio█

Freud (1969) studied children who █
mothers or families either at birth or du

These children consisted of orphans, war children, and certain concentration-camp children from Europe who grew up in England. In her work, Freud (1969) discussed some of the immediate effects of separation trauma:

- *Psychosomatic conditions:* feeding difficulties, sleep disturbances, constipation, and an increased propensity to develop sore throats or respiratory infections
- *Regression:* clinging, sucking, rocking, loss of speech, loss of impulse control, and loss of bowel and bladder control

The developmental functions that were most at risk were those which the children had most recently acquired.

Autonomy versus Shame and Doubt

During this developmental stage, the toddler sets out to achieve a sense of independence and learns a degree of self-restraint. This developmental feat is put in jeopardy, however, when the toddler witnesses adults around him or her engaging in violent acts, such as homicide, rape, and suicide. This type of behavior is hardly a model of self-restraint and, for the child, calls into question whether he or she can control his or her own aggressive impulses.

> No thing, perhaps, is more disillusioning to a child than becoming aware of a parent's attempted suicide or death by suicide. No other single parental act can so painfully accentuate issues of human accountability, the control of one's destructive impulses, or the child's dependence and helplessness. (Pynoos and Eth, 1985a, p. 35)

The impaired ability to control one's impulses is often noted in children who have been victims of physical and sexual abuse. In a study by George and Main (1979), hyperaggressive behavior was observed in infants and toddlers who had been physically abused. "Victims of physical abuse are typically unable to control aggression, while sexually abused children have difficulty containing and modulating sexual impulses" (Green, 1993, p. 579).

Competence in toilet training also occurs during this developmental stage as the toddler learns to regulate his or her own body by

"holding on" and "letting go" (Eriks(
with this accomplishment, however, b:
render the toddler helpless, thus causin
control and regress to a state of bed-v
pants.

Children who have witnessed the m
father, as well as the subsequent suicide
rienced a deterioration in their ability t
to master their own bodies (Pruett, 19
young children start feeling self-consci
ing them. "He would like to destroy the
must wish for his own invisibility" (Eri

Doubt is another negative consequei
sense of autonomy. Toddlers feel that t
therefore controlled by the will of other
lives in the hands of the very ones whc
This can be seen in cases of child abuse
tion, and child labor.

Initiative versus Guilt (Ages Three to .

During this stage, preschoolers deve
learn to initiate activities, pursue goal
They are also learning that not all behav
proval. They must achieve a balance bet
morally appropriate.

Preschoolers who are traumatized a
ment face the danger of feeling extreme
sies, and actions. According to Pruett (
"murderous fantasies, wishes, and fear
this developmental stage and "such chil
conflicted about, acting out the passiv
such fantasies."

Preschoolers who are traumatized at
their own sense of judgment. Those, for
abused, regardless of their actions, m;
themselves, and confused. They becor
fear of punishment.

Industry versus Inferiority (Ages Six to Twelve)

At this stage, school-age children learn to master various skills and earn recognition by becoming productive members of society. Through their successful completion of tasks, school-age children develop a sense of competence and personal satisfaction. An extreme stress and the feeling of helplessness that goes along with it, however, has a harmful effect on their perception of personal competence (Živčić, 1993).

School-age children who are traumatized may undergo a period of regression whereby newly mastered skills are no longer attainable. Failure to understand this lapse in ability may cause them to feel inadequate and inferior to their peers.

School age children who receive constant emotional abuse, for example, may not develop adequate self-esteem or confidence in their abilities. Instead of being rewarded for their successes, they are belittled and made to feel worthless. Being treated as an *Untermensch* (unworthy being) was more damaging for South African children living under apartheid than were the material deprivations (Silove and Schweitzer, 1993).

Identity versus Role Confusion (Ages Twelve to Eighteen)

During this stage, adolescents are "primarily concerned with what they appear to be in the eyes of others as compared with what they feel they are, and with the question of how to connect the roles and skills cultivated earlier with the occupational prototypes of the day" (Erikson, 1950, p. 261).

The adolescent who comes through this stage successfully develops a sense of identity, including a better knowledge of his or her place in society. Identity development is interrupted, however, when one is confused by the many complex roles that are present within society and decides to delay choosing a role, postponing adulthood altogether.

Adolescents who witness their mothers' rapes may choose to identify with the aggressor or with the victim. In a study of the transmission of war-related trauma, it was found that adolescents became more aggressive in their attempts to identify with their violent fathers. "This identification permits the child's fears of helplessness and anni-

hilation to be replaced by feelings of po\
ness, 1993, p. 639). In a study of childr
assault of their mothers, Pynoos and Na
adolescent who had planned to be an a
fantasies of becoming a gun merchant.

Following a traumatic experience, a
adopt a premature adult role. "The abru
nessing of violence may precipitate a pr
identity diffusions among adolescents'
Raundalen, 1993, p. 628).

Bolea and colleagues (2003) examin
of Sudanese refugee children. During c
to behave like adults to survive and th
United States, were expected to "regres
(p. 231).

How does a child who has been force
define his or her role in society? What
cents who have been traumatized by ar
the future. They have grown up in a wo
recognized childhood, so how then do
cence?

For adolescents who have been trau
something to fear, rather than to anticip
entering the workforce and return to
Kurdistan, Ahmad et al. (2000) noted tl
take on adult functions during times of d
increased their likelihood of further trau

MEMORY DEVELC

Infancy (Birth to Age Three)

The traumatized infant cannot trust in
tect his or her mother from sexual assau
cide—or which failed to protect him or
threat of abuse, or a severe natural disas
her has become terrifying, hostile, and ur
cumbs to a sense of basic mistrust, sham
would be better off, perhaps, if these earl

According to Cowan (1978), Piaget believed that the most significant thing that was absent in infants' tasks to make sense of the world around them was symbolic function. Newborns were incapable of holding onto images that would enable them to remember details of past events. They had no words, pictures, or gestures that they could draw upon in order to recall persons or objects, so that they could recollect events in their immediate present.

This ability to mentally represent images, according to Piaget, did not develop until the infant was able to achieve conceptual object permanence—the awareness that a person or thing still exists when out of sight (Cowan, 1978). To Piaget, it was not until the infant reached the age of about fifteen to twenty-four months that his or her sense of object permanence would be fully developed and he or she would begin to make vivid mental representations of people and events from the past. Further research studies contradicted Piaget's timing of several achievements and found that infants were able to conceptualize much earlier than was first believed. These findings are important when you consider the level of impact that traumatic experiences may have on infants.

Until recently, many people maintained a false assumption that infants were not affected by traumatic incidents because they were too young to be aware of or even remember what they had experienced. As infants progress through the first two years of life, however, behaviors appear that can only be attributed to memory. The second half of the first year appears to be a time of rapid growth in memory ability (Dacey and Travers, 1996). By the second half of the first year of life, infants not only exhibit the influence of earlier experiences through behaviors such as looking longer or kicking harder but also demonstrate the ability to recall specific events or episodes from their past— in some cases long after they occurred (Bauer, 1997).

By the end of the first year, infants can find hidden objects, and they can imitate actions of others hours or days after they first observed the behavior by the process of recall (remembering something that is not present). The beginnings of recall appear before the first year of age, as long as memories are strongly cued (Berk, 2000).

The organization of event representations and the availability of cues or reminders of to-be-remembered events have a profound impact on long-term memory in this age period (Bauer, 1997). As early as one and one-half to two years, children begin to talk about the past,

guided by adults who expand on th
(Berk, 2000).

Traumatic memories plague not onl
well, and they can be quite debilitatin
(1995) found that infants and toddlers (
velop posttraumatic disorders followir
who have experienced severe traumas
pairment, similar to posttraumatic syr
adults.

In their study of ninety toddlers wl
earthquake, Azarian et al. (1999) report
the youngest ones (ages ten to twenty-
earthquake), remembered the traumatic
place six months earlier. Their mem
verbally represented.

Preschoolers (Ages Three to Six)

Preschoolers are unable to think log
believing that the world revolves arou
clearly distinguish pretend from realit
deliberate in that they usually do not tr
instead, they remember events that ma
them (Papalia and Olds, 1993).

In a study of children's (ages three t
events, Goodman and colleagues (19⁹
was very high and children became nea
was associated with enhanced memor
(1995) found that some events which
age of three to four years may remain a
of five or six, and that some memories ⍳
early period even into adulthood.

School-Age Children and Adolescent.
(Ages Six to Eighteen)

School-age children are less egocen
logically. They are better at understa
space, as well as distinguishing reality

remember improves greatly during this time, and the amount of information they can remember increases (Papalia and Olds, 1993).

Adolescents during this developmental period, which Piaget referred to as formal operations, have the potential for "abstract understanding of motivation, alternative action, and the sequencing of events over a longer duration of time" (Pynoos and Eth, 1985b, p. 48). Adolescents are able to think abstractly and to acknowledge that in some situations there are no clear-cut answers.

"Having the cognitive maturity for deductive reasoning and the ability to understand the far-reaching consequences of a traumatic event, adolescents are in many ways more vulnerable to trauma exposure than are school-age children" (Macksoud, Dyregrov, and Raundalen, 1993, p. 628). Adolescents are quite capable of anticipating the personal impact that trauma will have on their lives. They no longer believe themselves to be invincible, unlike their younger counterparts (Pynoos and Eth, 1985b).

Certain trauma-related factors have a profound influence on children's memory. Following is a list of some of those factors mentioned by Pynoos and Nader (1989):

- Proximity to violence
- Perceptual experiences
- Distress signals
- Seeing victims
- Injury or blood
- Location and actions of adults
- Worry about a sibling
- Guilt
- Previous trauma

In a study of schoolchildren exposed to an Australian bushfire disaster, McFarlane (1987) reported that approximately one-third of the children had a continuing preoccupation with their exposure to the bushfire twenty-six months postdisaster. Children continued to dream about the fire, indicating the involuntary nature of their preoccupation.

In a survey of school-aged children three months after Hurricane Hugo, Lonigan et al. (1994) found that children who had a higher level of exposure (in terms of reported hurricane severity or home

damage) were most likely to experien
repetitive, intrusive, and upsetting thou
cane.

A great majority of children's memo
lenger explosion were consistent an
made by those of primary school age
than those of adolescents and may have
operational stage (Terr et al., 1996).

In a study of children (ages five to fo
the Chowchilla (California) school bus
ported that disturbances in cognitive fun
sense, and thought, occurred immediate
details of the kidnapping were remembe
incorrectly or ordered in the wrong se
the kidnapping (Terr, 1983) children'
mained intact and detailed.

TRAUMATIC FEARS (

Infants (Birth to Age Three)

Separation anxiety and stranger anx
by infants who have been traumatized. S
versally after the age of six months an
months (Berk, 2000). Separation anxie
has experienced prolonged separation
miliar caregivers due to a traumatic ir
Signs of separation anxiety include cli
ing left alone, difficulty sleeping, tan
Separation anxiety does not become di
emotions and behaviors have become
least a month (APA, 1994).

Separation anxiety was noted amon
Hurricane Hugo disaster (Saylor, Swens
toms included clinging to adults and
Clinging behavior and fear of being lef
toms observed in two- to six-year-olds
violence in South Africa (Dawes, Tred

Separation anxiety was observed in a seventeen-month-old infant who had been physically abused. Distress over the separation from the infant's mother persisted throughout the next year (Scheeringa et al., 1995).

The most frequent experience of fear during this period is stranger anxiety or fear of unfamiliar adults (Berk, 2000). Stranger anxiety is a normal fear of childhood but may become intensified during a trauma, especially when no parent or caretaker is available to offer comfort and security.

Preschoolers (Ages Three to Six)

Preschoolers have active imaginations and are, therefore, capable of developing many fears, such as fear of the dark, monsters on television, frightening noises, and dogs. It is also during this time that they have their first concerns regarding death (Schachter and McCauley, 1988).

Most fears of preschoolers tend to dissipate as they grow older. Those preschoolers who have been traumatized, however, live in a state of constant anxiety as fearful reminders of their negative experiences are triggered. Their fears, unfortunately, have been actualized and are no longer just figments of their overactive imaginations. They live in a world in which a parent *can* turn into a raging monster; bad things *do* occur in the dark; the sound of gunshots *is* a scary fact of life; and thunderstorms *can* evolve into life-threatening disasters, engulfing people and homes.

Elmer (1977) reported that the traumatized children in her study (victims of abuse and accidents) had "linked their fears of injury or mutilation to real persons, not fantasy figures. The other persons might be parents, older children, or school teachers" (pp. 276-277).

In a study of ten children (ages two to six years) who were allegedly sexually abused in a day care setting, Kiser and colleagues (1988) reported that many of the children reacted with "panic" behaviors to environmental stimuli related to their day care experiences. They were distressed by reminders such as passing the day care center or seeing one of the accused in the media.

Saylor, Swenson, and Powell (1992) examined parents' and preschoolers' reactions following Hurricane Hugo. Fear of water, refusal

to leave the parent, and unwillingness tc
problem behaviors parents reported am

School-Age Children (Ages Six to Tw

Passing fears are typical for school-ag
ing intelligence, they are more cognizai
danger. Fear of future attacks, fear of be
curity personnel were among the fears (
children whose communities had been
acts of political violence (Dawes, Trede

In a study of the impact of sexual al
sixteen), Wolfe, Gentile, and Wolfe (1!
ated fears were more prevalent among t
been sexually abused.

Girls who had survived the sinking c
and Murdoch, 1990) experienced a mul
of ships, swimming, water, the dark, ar

In a study of children of male polit
Philippines, Protacio-Marcelino (1989)
derwent extreme emotional stress due tc
perienced concerning the fate that mig
other problems. Nightmares, anxiety di
noises and sounds were among the prob
who survived a school pedestrian overp

Girls who witnessed the sexual assa
and Nader, 1988) became fearful of stra
neighborhoods. Children who survived tl
ing continued to worry about themselve
not feel safe (Pfefferbaum, Nixon, and

Adolescents (Ages Twelve to Eighteen

The number and severity of fears less
yield to feelings of anxiety, which can l
Epstein, and Stone, 1972). Anxiety ca
apprehensiveness, and generalized feeli
ficult to manage.

Following a traumatic incident, adol
rence of the trauma or that something h

Cambodian adolescent survivors of the Pol Pot regime displayed worries about friends, emotional withdrawal, and signs of anxiety over schoolwork (Sack et al., 1986). Nervousness and restlessness were among the most frequent posttraumatic stress reactions of displaced adolescents in Croatia (Ajdukovic, 1998).

CHILDREN'S UNDERSTANDING OF DEATH

Infants (Birth to Age Three)

According to Simpson (1993), infants and very young children sense death in nonverbal and noncognitive terms. Although they may not be able to verbally define death, they are familiar with it, are frightened by it, are inquisitive about it, and form lasting perceptions of it.

Children under the age of five do not perceive death as permanent. If a loved one dies, that person has simply gone away. The loved one's "departure" is not final. He or she continues to exist under other conditions (Schachter and McCauley, 1988).

Preschoolers (Ages Three to Six)

According to Yule, Perrin, and Smith (1999), children as young as four years old can have a partial or sometimes complete understanding of death. Without clear explanations, however, they attempt to understand death by relying on egocentric and magical thinking (Berk, 2000). Kane (1979), for example, reported that children in the beginning stage of developing a death concept believe that they can make someone dead by their own action, wish, or label. By the time children attend school (ages five to seven) they begin to demonstrate concepts of death similar to those of older children, relying less on magical thinking and more on biological and social reality (Swain, 1979).

School-Age Children (Ages Six to Twelve)

Younger school-age children (ages six to eight) do not quite understand the universality or the finality of death. According to Cuddy-Casey and Orvaschel (1997), however, most investigators have noted

a link between exposure to death and
some concepts of death among children
universality and finality. In a study of ch
ceptions of death and personal mortali
(1983) found that children who had suf
person were able to give more practical i
and the process of dying than those wh
tragedy.

Around age nine, school-age childre
to the point where they can comprehend
affects both young and old people. The
irreversible and final, but they still beli
people (Brooks and Siegel, 1996).

In a study of six- to ten-year-olds, Co
that conservation ability was more rela
rate concepts of death than was age. Orb
ported in their study of children ages te
the death concept appear to be independe
tioning.

Adolescents (Ages Twelve to Eighteen)

Adolescents are fully aware of the co
may perceive themselves as being invuln
in risk-taking behaviors, such as consu
hol, engaging in unprotected sex, and
adults, they are intrigued by death beca
them (Schachter and McCauley, 1988).

CULTURAL CONSID

The majority of children around the w
ditions that are very different from the I
middle-class standards of living, presup
and Olds,1993). Much of the research in
has focused on children in Western ind
quently, the standards that many mental I
identify problems in areas such as child c

ties, and child-rearing practices are largely those which reflect the majority culture (Coll and Meyer, 1993).

Identity and Self-Esteem

- In traditional African societies, individual self-esteem is not encouraged. The interests of the extended family or kinship group are of paramount concern and override the individual's interest (Nader, Dubrow, and Stamm, 1999).
- For Asian Americans, self-identity is closely related to ethnic identity. This tends to be less the case among white Americans (Chin, 1983).
- Due to their classification as ethnic minorities, refugee adolescents are in a marginal position. Losses such as career possibilities and social status pose a direct threat to their self-esteem and sense of identity (Van der Veer, 1998).
- Refugee adolescents have trouble establishing a strong sense of identity due to the traumatic experiences that destroyed most of the physical and emotional connections they had prior to the war (Lee, 1988).

Separation/Individuation

- In Chinese-American culture (e.g., practices of communal family sleeping arrangements and permissiveness in weaning), the concepts of early separation and individual privacy are regarded with less value in comparison to Western culture (Chin, 1983).
- One of the tasks in adolescence is to become less dependent, psychologically, on parents. This task is more challenging for those adolescents living in exile who haven't seen their parents for a period of years. "Contact with them was severed at a moment when the psychological process of separation and individuation, which occurs during adolescence, had not yet been completed" (Van der Veer, 1998, p. 219).
- American adolescents are expected to eventually move out of their parents' home and live on their own, whereas Southeast Asian youth tend to live in multigenerational households and are expected to take care of their parents until they die. The concept of separation thus poses a conflict with parental expectations and may lead to feelings of doubt and guilt among Southeast Asian refugee adolescents (Lee, 1988).

Future Orientation

- One of the many tasks of adolescenc
  cording to Van der Veer (1998), refug
  certain about their future. Any future
  tering exile was shattered by their
  with their self-image and worldview

  The adolescent has to learn to live
  possibilities he dreamed about are
  closed to him because the situati
  their realization and that the alter
  Veer, 1998, p. 220)

Child-Rearing Practices

- In Western culture, where the idea o
  ents is considered to be the norm, a tr
  ent, especially the mother who nour
  to be of great significance (Kareem.
  cultures, however, the mother-child
  than the sibling-child dyad, the cov
  mother-child dyad. There may be nc
  the primary caregiver (Wilson-Oyela
  of loss consists of a much broader sp
  one individual parent exists. Loss is
  relations: "the loss of their roots, of
  ment, and of the memories of mul
  2000, p. 29).
- Harmonious family relationships are
  tional cultures, such as Nigeria. In an
  of relationships within the extended
  ment of loyalty to the biological pa
  preference for solidarity with the la
  1989, p. 56). A series of behavioral
  are, therefore, devised to allay the ef
  ents (Wilson-Oyelaran, 1989).

SUMMARY

1. The infant (birth to age three) learns to develop a sense of basic trust—the willingness to let mother out of sight without undue anxiety or rage because she has become an inner certainty and an outer predictability (Erikson, 1950).
2. The impaired ability to control one's impulses is often noted in children who have been victims of physical and sexual abuse.
3. The school-age child who has been traumatized may undergo a period of regression in which newly mastered skills are no longer attainable.
4. Following a traumatic experience, adolescents may be forced to adopt a premature adult role.
5. Traumatic memories plague adults and the very young, and they can be quite debilitating.
6. Fivush, Haden, and Adam (1995) found that some events which were experienced before the age of three to four years may remain accessible, at least until the age of five or six, and that some memories may be retained from this very early period even into adulthood.
7. The ability to remember improves greatly during school age, and the amount of information remembered also increases (Papalia and Olds, 1993).
8. "Having the cognitive maturity for deductive reasoning and ability to understand the far-reaching consequences of a traumatic event, adolescents are in many ways more vulnerable to trauma exposure than are school-age children" (Macksoud, Dyregrov, and Raundalen, 1993, p. 628).
9. Separation anxiety and stranger anxiety are frequently expressed by infants who have been traumatized.
10. Preschoolers who have been traumatized live in a state of constant anxiety as fearful reminders of their negative experiences are triggered.
11. The number and severity of fears lessen as children grow older and yield to feelings of anxiety, which can be more detrimental (Landau, Epstein, and Stone, 1972).
12. Children under the age of five do not perceive death as permanent (Schachter and McCauley, 1988).

13. According to Cuddy-Casey and O
    gators have noted a link between e>
    understanding of some concepts o
    age seven, particularly universality
14. Adolescents are fully aware of the
    they may perceive of themselves a
    (Schachter and McCauley, 1988).
15. Universal aspects of child developr
    ships across ethnic and cultural g
    mented.

Chapter 3

How Children Respond
to Traumatic Incidents

> Rwandans fleeing the mass killing in their village are emotion-
> ally numb by the time they reach the border with Zaire. A Viet-
> nam War veteran abuses alcohol and cannot hold down a job. A
> child becomes withdrawn and takes no interest in her school-
> work after her family is forced to move to a homeless shelter.
> Across national borders, people who have been traumatized
> share many of the same symptoms. (Crosby and Van Soest, 1997,
> p. 47)

It is difficult to fathom that, following a traumatic incident, children (from infancy through adolescence) are capable of experiencing
the same level of emotional pain and horror as adults. It may seem
easier to adopt the belief that most children are resilient by nature and
quickly forget about any negative experiences they may have encountered on their road to adulthood. If only this were true.

Unfortunately, children are not able to escape traumatic experiences unscathed. The support of family, friends, and community does
help a great deal, but it is not always available or sufficient. As a result, children learn to cope with the trauma the best way they know
how (e.g., with denial, regression, acting out, avoidance, or identification with the aggressor).

Traumatized children may appear on the surface to be holding up
quite well. If we were to look closer, however, we might notice that
many of these children are in so much pain that no words can describe
it. The only way they may be able to tell us is by their own behavior,
such as having difficulty sleeping, expressing intense fear of separation or strangers, acting younger, being easily frustrated, not wanting
to be left alone, having difficulty concentrating, and/or showing loss
of appetite. These are just a few of the possible indicators of post-

traumatic stress to which we are all vu
toms worsen over time, however, a
emerge: post-traumatic stress disorder.

Millions of children are suffering fro
new and chilling term in the internation
is considered to be the most prevalei
health condition; it may follow exposi
which there is the presence of real or in
or the risk of grave physical injury to
others.

It was not until 1980 that PTSD becai
diagnostic category of anxiety disorder
to be a disorder found only in combat v
widely known and accepted that PTSI
traumatic incidents, particularly those
can affect children and adults, males
dents that can trigger PTSD include vic
armed conflict, homicide, suicide, sexu;

Once PTSD occurs, the severity ar
vary. Symptoms of PTSD may be delay
at any moment following the initial trau
clude intrusions such as nightmares as
sive behaviors. If these symptoms per
may develop into acute PTSD. Sympton
and beyond may develop into chronic P'
an onset of symptoms at least six mont.
dent.

COMMON POSTTRAUN
REACTIONS OF C.

I believe that PTSD, in children anc
sponse to a very primal loss of inno
with the irreversibility of some ki
1993, p. 619)

Several studies (Scheeringa and Zea
Saylor, Swenson, and Powell, 1992; S

1995; McFarlane, 1987; Pynoos and Nader, 1988; Shaw et al., 1995; Goldstein, Wampler, and Wise, 1997; Terr, 1981b; Pynoos et al., 1987; Nader et al., 1990; Lonigan et al., 1994; Shannon et al., 1994; Giaconia et al., 1995; Ajdukovic, 1998) report the presence of symptoms that seem specific to children's reactions to trauma. These symptoms are described in the following sections according to age group.

Infants and Toddlers (Birth to Age Three)

- *Fear*—Fear is a common experience following a traumatic incident. Infants and toddlers are especially prone to fearful emotions and behaviors, due to their limited understanding of life events. Typical fears in this age group are separation and stranger anxiety.
- *Hyperarousal*—Infants and toddlers may become easily aroused or have startle reactions (involuntary trembling, jumpiness, or tensing of the muscles) to noises, such as a fire engine, a police siren, or thunder, which remind them of their traumatic experiences. Sudden movements (such as a falling object or person running toward them) can also trigger startle reactions.
- *Aggression*—Temper tantrums, kicking, biting, screaming, and lashing out are all ways that infants and toddlers may respond following a traumatic incident. These behaviors communicate the frustration, fear, or confusion that they feel on the inside but are not able to express verbally.
- *Sleep difficulties*—Many children in this age group have difficulty sleeping following a traumatic incident due to night terrors, fear of sleeping alone, nightmares, etc.
- *Clinging*—Traumatized infants and toddlers may cling to their parents or caretakers out of an extreme need to feel safe and protected. Because of a fear of separation, strangers, or other traumatic reminders, they may not want to be left alone for even a moment, and it is not uncommon for them to want to be held constantly for reassurance that they will not be abandoned.
- *Easily frustrated*—Children in this age group have a tendency to become easily frustrated when there are sudden, unexpected changes in their environment and when the people they have come to trust and rely upon no longer seem trustworthy or reliable, at least in their eyes.

- *Regression*—Newly discovered skill
  traumatic experience. For example, to
  may revert to soiling their pants or
  could speak fairly well may suddenl
  attempts of the traumatized infant or
  of trauma.
- *Whining*—Children become increasi
  overwhelmed following a traumatic
  their emotions at this age, they resor
  can be quite trying for some parent
  overwrought themselves.
- *Irritability*—Traumatized infants and
  cranky than usual and are difficult to
  fussing is common.

Preschoolers (Ages Three to Six)

- *Reenactment of the incident*—Traum
  enact themes or aspects of their tra
  such as having action figures repeate
  ing a house of blocks and knocking
  planes into the ground. These are all
  their experiences and a sense of relie
  tressful, however, that no relief is obt
  out the trauma, the more helpless the
- *Regression*—Like infants and toddle
  tendency to regress following a trau
  resort to such behaviors as thumb su
  to sleep alone.
- *Clinging*—Preschoolers who have been
  in dependency, and they need reassur
  their lives are not going to abandon th
  fend for themselves. They may resort
  to feel safe again and obtain some lev
- *Insecurity*—Preschoolers may feel the
  shattered as a result of their traumatic
  will ever be the same again. They loo
  to restore their sense of security.

- *Anger*—Traumatic incidents that occur with no explanation or one that is difficult to comprehend can result in the preschooler feeling angry. This anger can be so intense that it often leads to aggressive behavior.
- *Temper tantrums*—Preschoolers have limited verbal capacities. When frustrated, they may resort to having temper tantrums rather than verbally expressing how they feel.
- *Fear*—The normal fears of preschoolers can be exacerbated following a traumatic experience. Fear of the dark, thunderstorms, death, separation, and strangers can become extreme and obsessive.
- *Sleep disturbances*—Following a traumatic experience, preschoolers may have disturbed sleep patterns. This can be attributed to nightmares, intense fear, sleepwalking, etc.

School-Age Children (Ages Six to Twelve)

- *Separation anxiety*—Traumatized children of this age group may refuse to leave one or both parents due to fear of something horrible happening to them, such as an illness, disaster, or death. This fear is typical in school-age children but is intensified in those who have undergone a traumatic experience. Separation anxiety of this magnitude may lead to avoidance of social activities and refusal to attend school.
- *Guilt*—Traumatic experiences often result in associated feelings of guilt among this age group. They may blame themselves for not being able to offer assistance; for having survived when others lost their lives; or for having done something that caused others to be harmed.
- *Clinging*—Clinging is one form of regressive behavior that occurs among traumatized school-age children. They may have a desire to hold onto a security object that they used to have when younger, such as a favorite blanket or stuffed animal. They may also hover around their parents, refusing to let them out of their sight for fear that they may disappear.
- *Diminished interest in activities*—Traumatized children may feel depressed, overwhelmed, anxious, or confused and, as a result, show a lack of desire to engage in activities. They are unable to find enjoyment in those things that used to be pleasurable, such as play-

ing games, participating in sports,
television.

- *Reenactment of the trauma in pla*
  pretend that they are reliving their t
  this in the form of play and may act
  but in reality they are quite distresse
  and may be reckless or even danger
  trol over the trauma which left them
- *Reduced impulse control*—Traumatiz
  sively by lashing out at their parents
  ing property, etc. If they have witne
  an out-of-control manner, children c
  own ability to "hold it all together."
- *Physical complaints* (e.g., headache
  a traumatic experience, school-age c
  aches, dizziness, stomach pains, d
  physical ailments. There appears to
  their symptoms, but they are "real"
  caused by extreme stress.
- *Avoidance*—School-age children ma
  attempt to avoid anything, any plac
  might remind them of their traumatic
  havior may hamper daily activities
  and school performance. It may al
  tranged and alone. Fear of separati
  cism, and reaction may also lead to
  children.
- *Intrusive thoughts, images, and sou*
  ages, and sounds often torment scho
  traumatized. These intrusions can
  time (e.g., during conversation, at b
  house). The intrusions are triggered
  ment, such as a neighborhood street,
  reactions of others, and can lead t
  scribed earlier.
- *Recurrent distressing dreams*—Tra
  group often have distressing dreams
  the night or for many nights. These d
  of the trauma and may interfere with

- *Hypervigilance*—School-age children who have been traumatized may become quite vigilant to what they perceive as danger in their environment. They are easily startled and react with nervousness or jumpiness.
- *Fear of further trauma*—School-age children often fear a recurrence of the trauma. As a result, they are always on guard, hoping that they will be better prepared for the next traumatic incident. These children live as if they are on a minefield, waiting for the next bomb to explode. This type of fear can become an obsession, occupying the majority of their time.
- *Sadness*—School-age children can feel a pervasive sense of sadness following a traumatic incident. They may have suffered great loss and feel very lonely. Withdrawal, tearfulness, and loss of interest in previously enjoyed activities may ensue.
- *Regression*—Regression is common among traumatized children in this age group. It is one way of coping with their negative experiences. They may become more dependent; express temper tantrums, whining, and clinging behaviors; and refuse to sleep alone. There may also be a return to thumb sucking, bed-wetting, and soiling accidents.
- *Sleep disturbances*—The sleep patterns of children are often disrupted by a traumatic experience. They may have difficulty falling asleep, have early morning awakenings, or sleep excessively. Nightmares, intrusive images and thoughts, night terrors, bed-wetting, and sleepwalking all contribute to sleep deprivation and disturbances.
- *Sense of foreshortened future*—Traumatized children may feel helpless and insecure about their future. They sometimes try to tempt fate by engaging in reckless and dangerous behavior.
- *Difficulty paying attention*—Traumatized children may have difficulty concentrating or focusing on tasks, especially schoolwork. They often appear lethargic, as though they have little or no energy.
- *Difficulty trusting*—Traumatized children may perceive the world to be an unsafe place and, therefore, feel the need to fend for themselves in order to survive. The sense of security and trust that they have in significant others may be altered by their negative experiences and may be difficult to reestablish.
- *Decrease in school performance*—Intrusions, preoccupation with the traumatic event, difficulty concentrating, lack of sleep, and low

energy all interfere with the schoc
children. They may not learn as mt
class; have difficulty getting along v
extracurricular activities; or have c
tasks.

Adolescents (Ages Twelve to Eightee.

* *Dreams of the incident*—Adolescents
  in their dreams, which too often turn
  tend to interfere with sleep, causing
  edly during the night. The dreams ⅰ
  recur for years.
* *Avoidance*—Adolescents who have
  draw from family and friends. They ⅰ
  periences or participate in social ac
  adolescents choose to avoid traumaⅰ
  hol and drugs.
* *Guilt*—Traumatized adolescents m₂
  ing able to intervene effectively to ⅰ
  may believe that perhaps they co
  change the results of what happenec
  negative self-image.
* *Sense of foreshortened future*—Ad
  mistic about the future following a t
  high-risk behaviors (e.g., promiscui
  abuse) because of a feeling of disill
  their future is limited. Traumatize
  nessed how fragile life can be may ⅰ
  ture. This feeling of hopelessness
  and/or behaviors.
* *Diminished interest in activities*—'
  feel depressed and show a lack of iⅰ
  ously enjoyed. They may appear to b
  themselves.
* *Hypervigilance*—Traumatized adolⅰ
  stantly wary and suspicious of othe
  are sometimes easily agitated by exte
  tions may be perceived as hostile.

- *Intrusive imagery* (e.g., flashbacks)—Sights, sounds, smells, and other triggers associated with memories of the traumatic experience can resurface in adolescents. They may feel as if the trauma is happening all over again and thus become terrified.
- *Difficulty concentrating*—Traumatized adolescents often have difficulty concentrating. Intrusive images, for example, may cause their minds to wander. Schoolwork is put in jeopardy as a result of their difficulty focusing on tasks that require extended attention.
- *Difficulty sleeping*—Traumatized adolescents often have difficulty falling and staying asleep. Their nightmares can be intense and repetitive.
- *Emotional numbing*—Adolescents may attempt to detach themselves emotionally in an effort to avoid feeling retraumatized. They may be seen daydreaming and fantasizing, which interferes with their ability to concentrate.
- *Appetite disturbances*—Traumatized adolescents may develop appetite disturbances, such as overeating or loss of appetite, to help defend themselves against painful emotions and intrusive recollections associated with their trauma. Overeating, refusal to eat, and other appetite disturbances may be an attempt by adolescents to gain some sense of control over their traumatic experiences. Eating disorders, such as anorexia and bulimia, may emerge as a result.
- *Depression*—Extreme sadness, helplessness, and pessimism about the future, a pervasive sense of loss, excessive guilt and shame—all may lead to depression in adolescents.
- *Anger*—Feelings of anger, irritability, and rage are often present in traumatized adolescents. They may have uncontrollable outbursts of temper, resulting in destruction of property and hostility toward others. Social relations can be negatively affected, as a result.
- *Problems with alcohol and drugs*—Traumatized adolescents may experiment with drugs and alcohol to avoid intrusive recollections and to numb the emotional pain that they feel. Such behavior can result in cognitive impairment, reckless behavior, and substance abuse.
- *Pregnancy*—Adolescents may engage in sexual promiscuity and unsafe sexual practices in an effort to shield themselves against the anxiety associated with traumatic recollections. This sexual acting-out behavior may result in unwanted pregnancies and sexually transmitted diseases.

- *Suicidal thoughts and attempts*—T
  feel hopeless and depressed, and n
  drawn. Seeing no end to their sufferi
  of suicide. They often do not wish to
  may lead to attempted, or even comp
- *Somatic complaints*—Adolescents fo
  report headaches, dizziness, breathin
  and other somatic complaints. Upon
  planation may be found.

SPECIFIC P.
AND STRESS-RESPONSE-RE

Reenactment in Play

> Whereas an ordinary child can co
> that there will be a happy ending,
> differently. No happy endings are
> play ending must be repeated aga
> satisfying. The child hopes that the
> (Terr, 1981a, p. 757)

Preschool and school-age children w
matic incidents often engage in reenact
incident. Reenactment in play may inv
forts at mastery, identification with th
seek revenge or validate the traumatic o
Sugar (1988) examined the effects o
boy who had been exposed to an airpla
ence of reenactment. The boy used toy a
play out the crash. Terr (1981b) studie
five to fourteen) five to thirteen months
in a school bus kidnapping. She found
kidnapping behaviors that were direc
fears, or actions which had occurred be
The repeated reenactments accounted 1
school performance, psychophysiologi
ing anxiety in several of the kidnapped

Saylor, Swenson, and Powell (1992) studied parents' observations of their preschoolers' play in the year following Hurricane Hugo. One child's reenactment of the trauma involved the use of broccoli spears at dinner, which he used to represent trees being ravaged again and again; another child played the role of a roofer who repaired a house.

Reenactment in play was noted in children who were victims of an earthquake in Italy (Galante and Foa, 1986). The children played the "earthquake" game, whereby the lives of everyone were destroyed. They would shake the table to simulate the rumble of the earthquake.

Intrusive Imagery

> How can you get this picture out of your mind? How can you forget that your sister was repeatedly raped, stabbed, or strangled? How can you concentrate on the history of World War II without thinking of violence and destruction and imagine the face of your killed brother or sister? (Kübler-Ross, 1997, p. 105)

People who suffer from PTSD may continue to reexperience the traumatic incident in their minds. These reexperiences can take place in the form of intrusive imagery such as flashbacks, nightmares, unwelcomed thoughts, disruptive images, and terrifying, graphic illusions about the incident. A child's reexperiences can be noticed in play, artwork, discussions with peers, dreams of being a superhero and rescuing others, life threat to self or others, and nightmares of scary monsters.

Triggers are part of the reexperiencing phenomenon made manifest by those who suffer from PTSD. These unwelcomed occurrences are generally unpredictable and take place without warning. Despite knowledge of their unreality, these reactions are experienced as real. Some common triggers include the following:

- Sound (e.g., thunder, sirens, gunshots, screams, helicopters)
- Smell (e.g., ashes, gas, alcohol)
- Touch (e.g., a hug or kiss on the cheek)
- Specific sights (e.g., a familiar color, a foggy day, a full moon, water)
- Movement (e.g., someone running behind an individual or jumping in front of him or her)
- Situational (e.g., being afraid, feeling helpless)

- Stories or conversations about topi
  cidents
- Media (e.g., television, newspaper:
  tional, the subject matter may ind
  triggers

Three months after Hurricane Hugo,
a higher level of exposure in terms of
damage were most likely to experience s
petitive, intrusive, and upsetting thought
(Lonigan et al., 1994). Six months after I
of children whose homes were floode
experiencing the event (Russoniello et a
Nader et al. (1990) did a fourteen-m
children involved in the sniper attack ar
ery remained prominent for the most dir
described continued thoughts and imag
jured and bleeding classmates, bullets s
sounds of gunfire, and cries for help.
Intrusive images were the most freq
among displaced adolescents in Croatia
who witnessed murder of a parent experi
homicidal scene (e.g., knife wounds ir
quist, 1986). The intrusive recollection
such as during the middle of conversatic

Sleep Disturbances

Traumatized children often remember
not only while awake but also during sle
dreams, nightmares, insomnia, episodes
asleep, or fear of sleeping alone. The t
bered and relived during sleep, even tho
what he or she was actually dreaming al
Glod and Teicher (1996) examined th
physical and sexual abuse, PTSD, and ac
children. They found that the abused ch
bedtime and had a prominent period of a
et al. (1987) found that among the highl

in a sniper attack, dreams depicting the attack were frequent and accompanied by a renewed feeling of intense life threat.

Since the Buffalo Creek flood disaster in 1972, Newman (1976) has described one preschooler who screamed in his sleep and another preschooler who often slept with his mother in the same bed and desired to be rocked. Children involved in a school bus kidnapping continued to have repetitive nightmares four years later. Those who dreamed primarily "unremembered terror dreams" tended to talk or walk in their sleep (Terr, 1983, p. 1547).

Somatic Complaints

Somatic complaints, such as chest pain, stomachaches, and headaches, are often reported among traumatized children of all ages. Pynoos and Nader (1988) conducted a study of children who witnessed the sexual assault of their mothers. Some made complaints of recurring nausea and feeling ill more often. School-age children appeared to be more susceptible to minor infections, and physical injuries were noted among the older adolescents due to accident proneness and frequent physical altercations.

Headaches, stomach pains, and dizziness were among the complaints of children who witnessed parental murder (Malmquist, 1986). One boy suffered prolonged diarrhea (for two months) following a parental murder. No medical explanation was found.

Hypervigilance

Hypervigilance is excessive alertness. The body goes into a self-protective mode and prepares itself for flight. Internally displaced Bosnian children felt as if they were once again amid hostilities just by being in the presence of military personnel and hearing loud noises (Goldstein, Wampler, and Wise, 1997).

Deprivation was associated with significantly increased symptoms of hypervigilance in children and adolescents during siege conditions in Sarajevo (Husain et al., 1998). Hypervigilance and an exaggerated startle response was noted in a five-month-old infant with cancer (Roy and Russell, 2000).

Avoidant Responses

This set of responses involves effor
people, situations, activities, or discuss
matic incident. The child's peer relatio
as he or she withdraws socially to avc
dent.

Children who are feeling overwhelr
certain people, sounds, smells, places
incident) tend to become isolated, find
can often be seen daydreaming. As a re:
pear disoriented, elusive, indifferent, r
and they may act as if nothing is botheri
as if in another world.

> Psychic numbing may become a v
> acter flaw. The person who lives
> pression, beyond feeling, will pr
> The absent eyes, the blunted res;
> these vacancies frighten anyone '
> ally mean. Who lives behind the
> many times—an ordinary child
> p. 94)

Children who were screened for PT:
lowing a school shooting reported feel
lacked interest in significant activities (;
Children who had been allegedly sexua
(Kiser et al., 1988) refused to see their
actions that in any way evoked though
Adolescents who reported being rap
show symptoms of avoidance in a stud;
(1995).

Foreshortened Future

Traumatized children may experienc
pessimism about the future. According
tation is important in helping childrer
their socialization to adult roles. It guic

prepares them for what may lie ahead in their future (e.g., marriage, employment, parenthood, retirement). Trauma jeopardizes future orientation, thus causing children to feel a sense of hopelessness and pessimism concerning their futures.

Some observers have noted a pattern of "terminal thinking" among those most affected by trauma: "Terminal thinking is most clearly evident when, in response to the question, 'what do you expect to be when you are 30 years old?' the youth answers, 'Dead'" (Garbarino, 1999, pp. 171-172).

Internally displaced Bosnian children showed extreme pessimism regarding their future when they reported that they believed they would never be happy and felt that life was not worth living (Goldstein, Wampler, and Wise, 1997). Four years following the kidnapping of their school bus, twenty-three of twenty-five victims suffered from severe "philosophical pessimism," the sense that their futures would be extremely limited (Terr, 1983, p. 1547).

Guilt

Following a traumatic incident, children may feel guilty for having survived or being unable to offer assistance. Children exposed to a fatal sniper attack on their school playground (Pynoos et al., 1987) reported "feeling bad" about being unable to provide aid, being safe when others were harmed, or taking actions that they believe harmed others. These expressions of guilt were associated with severe posttraumatic reaction. Guilt over acts of omission and/or commission believed to have caused harm to others was the most severe symptom reported by children exposed to an earthquake in Armenia (Goenjian et al., 1995).

Anger

Anger may not only reflect the hyperarousal state associated with posttraumatic reactions but also may be a response to the chaos brought on by the many disruptions and changes that take place during the aftermath of a traumatic incident. Irritability and anger were common responses among children who witnessed the sexual assault of their mothers (Pynoos and Nader, 1988) and resulted in reduced

tolerance of the normal behaviors of th
ness to respond with aggression.

Decline in School Performance

Following a traumatic incident, chil
perience a decline in their school perfor
found in their study that adolescents
lower high school grade point averages
matized.

A significant drop occurred in the
mances of children exposed to Hurr.
1994). Cambodian adolescent survivor
et al., 1986) displayed anxiety over sc
signs of daydreaming and emotional w

Separation Anxiety

Separation anxiety manifests itself
the parent in order to attend school or c
fear that some disaster will happen if h
parent (Schachter and McCauley, 1988
One and a half years after an earth
et al. (1995) found that symptoms of s
sive among children throughout the e
boy exposed to a plane crash disaster (
felt insecure, and exhibited increased s
Of the trauma-related characteristics
(1991) suggests four that seem to endu
trusive imagery, reenactments, trauma
foreshortened future.

TERRORISM AND W.
REACTIONS AND S

Reactions

Following the terrorist attacks of Se
forts were made by trauma experts and

to assist caregivers who work with children in the identification of trauma symptoms and the application of emergency response procedures. Educators were expected to explain to children the horrific events that had taken place and to identify those students who were at risk. Counselors were called upon to offer debriefing sessions and strategies for coping with the tragedy. Parents were encouraged to talk with their children about their feelings and to be supportive. What an enterprise!

Government officials from ten countries—Canada, France, Japan, Israel, Mexico, Ireland, Spain, Turkey, United Kingdom, and the United States—met in Washington, DC, to discuss strategies for helping schools prepare for and respond to terrorist attacks. Those in the helping profession had little information to draw upon, since no event of this nature had been thoroughly researched or studied in reference to children's reactions—with the exception of, perhaps, the Oklahoma City bombing in 1995.

Lists of posttraumatic stress symptoms that children exhibit and various coping strategies based on earlier trauma research were quickly distributed to U.S. schools, as well as uploaded and downloaded throughout cyberspace. All of this information is needed and helpful. However, an important distinction must be made. The effects of trauma, stemming from acts of terrorism and war, are usually far more complex, severe, and chronic than those of single-event traumas such as an automobile accident or an apartment fire.

Survivors of war and terrorism carry lifelong emotional and physical scars that are capable of wounding not just individuals but whole societies and cultures for generations to come. Silver and Rogers (2002) best describe the nature of war and terrorist trauma in their book, titled *Light in the Heart of Darkness: EMDR and the Treatment of War and Terrorism Survivors.*

Unlike single-event trauma, terrorism and war trauma typically involve a series of horrifying events (Silver and Rogers, 2002). As in the case of terrorism, there is the threat and/or reality of repeated attacks, counterterrorism, economic losses, ongoing court trials, endlessly repeated media images of destruction, and continued loss of loved ones as bodies are recovered and those who lay ill in the hospital take their final breaths.

War causes incidents of displacement, malnutrition, disease, rape, torture, land mine casualties, ensuing threats of violence, as well as

loss of family members, support syste
sources. Any one of these events woul

What child who has lived in a countr
siege of terrorism has not witnessed ca
speakable pain? Millions of children
real-life horror films: depicting execut
body parts strewn everywhere, and thre
cera being splattered on the pavement b
that they hear are actual bombs being de
These children are forced to view and
posed to be "for adults only." While co
of terrorism remains imminent, these
encing further pain and suffering as
shown repeatedly on television. Many
deep and lasting psychological scars.

The traumatic experiences of war a
ending. The ongoing conflict between
ians, after all, has its origins in the Old T
no peaceful resolution has been foun
volved in civil war since the 1970s, and
dren continue to endure hardship and li
tainty.

One other distinguishing aspect of v
cording to Silver and Rogers (2002), is
carry. Traumas such as natural disasters
God," whereas war and terrorism trau
Survivors may question God for allowi
even though God is not the one setting
the airplanes, carrying out the execution
ture. On the other hand, knowing that
sponsible for such atrocities has an adde
of the world, understanding of relatic
means to be human.

Silver and Rogers (2002) describe a
rorism trauma that they refer to as the e
happens to other people. Children in Si
ern Uganda, for example, were forced
bers being tortured and murdered, and t
peated bombings and explosives (UNIC

Drawings by Palestinian children who grew up in the Infitada depicted children being beaten or shot by soldiers (Garbarino, Kostelny, and Dubrow, 1991). This kind of trauma is typically repetitive in nature, and just living in a particular place, according to Silver and Rogers (2002), can greatly enhance the probability of being exposed to more than one traumatic event:

> A war refugee does not see something bad happen to others once, but many times. Particularly in limited geographical areas, such as a town or city under the siege of terrorism, a person is likely to encounter multiple scenes of carnage. (Silver and Rogers, 2002, p. 15)

Children who are victims of war and terrorism include not just those who are injured or killed in the violence but also those who are survivors, relatives, witnesses, bystanders, and other civilians. A quarter of a million children were slaughtered during the 1994 genocide in Rwanda. Kosovar children were forced from their homes and uprooted from everything familiar to them during the ethnic cleansing that occurred in 1999. Children witnessed adults jumping out of windows as high as the 80th floor during the September 11, 2001, attacks on the World Trade Center in the United States.

Children across the globe suffer from posttraumatic stress symptoms associated with their experiences of war and terrorism. These symptoms bear some similarities to those of other traumas:

- The *New England Journal of Medicine* conducted a survey of stress reactions following the terrorist attacks that occurred in New York on September 11, 2001. They found that 35 percent of parents reported that their children experienced difficulty sleeping, difficulty concentrating, irritability, and nightmares. Forty-seven percent of parents reported that their children were worried about their own safety or the safety of a loved one (Schuster et al., 2001).
- Middle and high school students in the Oklahoma City public schools were surveyed following the 1995 bombing of the Alfred P. Murrah Federal Building. They reported having the following symptoms at the time of the explosion: psychological arousal, helplessness, perceived life threat, and concerns for the safety of family members and friends (Pfefferbaum et al., 1999).

- Children whose parents were killed i
  viewed ten years following the incide
  of three out of four children was ch;
  control, pessimism, reenactment be
  problems, antisocial behavior, and in
  lems (Dreman and Cohen, 1990).
- A study of Lebanese preschool child
  exposure to heavy shelling during a
  major behavioral problems: refusal
  dependence on parents, excessive th
  (Zahr, 1996).
- In a study of Guatemalan Mayan
  government-sponsored terrorism (di
  population from 1981 to 1983), it w
  fear continued to haunt the children
  terrorism five to seven years previous
  gest felt emotion by both children in
  ville and Lykes, 1992).

Symptoms

For the mental health clinician, the r
are indistinguishable.

Anger

Anger is an emotional aftereffect that
ger is directed externally against the te
having done more to prevent the incider
ing of insecurity over having lost pers
Their victimization could rob them of
(Mullins, 1997).

Guilt

When others are injured or perisl
wonder why. The need to believe i
great that, rather than abandon th
judge himself or herself as having
thereby survived. (Silver and Rog

Many victims of terrorism feel guilty for having survived when members of their families or friends perished. They may feel a sense of failure and a desire to avenge their deaths. Being called to testify may rekindle these feelings of guilt.

Fear

Many victims of terrorism are terrified of darkness, strangers, and changes in environment, and have pronounced startle responses to loud noises or sudden movement. The threat of terrorism can persist and may result in debilitating anxiety and phobic reactions. Also, new terrorist activities, court trials of terrorists, and related events may precipitate latent anxieties.

Difficulty Sleeping

A child who has been the victim of war or terrorism would find it very difficult to sleep. Nightmares, restlessness, and fear of the dark are all common. The problem becomes compounded when a child has to sleep amid hostilities and the sounds of explosives, gunfire, and cries in the dark. When a child is forced to sleep in the crowded, unsafe conditions of a refugee camp, he or she may be subject to rape and other abuses. So the question becomes, Does one even dare to sleep?

Difficulty Concentrating

Some acts of terrorism happen adjacent to school buildings or even on school property. Children are expected to return to school and resume their work as usual after having been debriefed and counseled. How does one concentrate when the bloodstains are still visible on the floors; the bullet holes remain etched in the walls; and haunting sounds of panic can be heard echoing through the corridors? For many victims of terrorism, the ability to focus and concentrate becomes a tumultuous task, especially when the media serves as a constant reminder of their traumatic experience.

Hypervigilance

Children who live in war zones have a heightened sense of vigilance. They have become like the soldiers around them—always on

guard for the first sign of danger. It
leaves, or a faint whisper. The slightes
beat, cause beads of perspiration to fo
send a wave of panic throughout the b
nals that the enemy is fast approachin₃

Alcohol and Drug Abuse

Alcohol and drugs are sometimes us
ing for victims of ongoing suffering.
adults attempting to alleviate their suf
see no harm in doing the same. The ris
and even death becomes a harsh realit

Aggression

Anger that is unresolved can result
Identification with the aggressor is con
up amid armed conflict, especially whe
martyr or a victim of an unjust society

Flashbacks

Long after a terrorist attack or act of
ages remain and can awaken memorie:
in the form of flashbacks. Flashbacks
sensory system that has the strongest
smoky odor; body bags lined up on the
shouts of evacuation; people caked in
clouds of noxious smoke; the smell of
about; or the frantic cries of families ar
amples. These images are quite familia
bombing of the World Trade Center on
thereafter. After the rubble has all been
ers lurk around the corner until they c;

Concern for Safety

The experience and the continued th
a way of shaking one's sense of securit

does one feel safe after witnessing the execution or torture of family members and friends; whole communities being burned to the ground; years of violence, illness, famine, and homelessness? A wave of uncertainty is a constant fixture in the lives of children whose lives have been torn apart by armed conflict. They have suffered unrecoverable losses.

Helplessness

A sense of helplessness seems almost inevitable among children who have witnessed atrocities that would weaken the stomachs of the most hardened adults. What little power children may have is all stripped away when their families, communities, and nations come under siege. The very adults who are supposed to protect them have fallen before them.

Reenactment Behavior

Reenactment in play may be a way for children to validate and obtain mastery over their traumatic experiences. It may also be a way to identify with the aggressor or a cry for help or revenge.

> In the West Bank's Jalazon refugee camp, Palestinian children play the game of Infitada. The children playing the part of the Palestinian demonstrators gather stones to throw at the children playing the part of Israeli soldiers. The soldiers then charge the demonstrators, hitting them with sticks, "firing" tear gas canisters, and shooting them with stick guns. Sometimes children really do get hurt when they are hit with a stone or poked with a stick. All this, when in the real world more than 50,000 children—about 1 in every 20 Palestinian children—have been seriously injured in the real-life "limited war" in which they live. (Garbarino, Kostelny, and Dubrow, 1991, p. 12)

Regression

Regression is a normal defensive tool that is readily accessible to children during times of stress. The behaviors associated with regression tend to last for only a short period of time and are reversible. However, children who have been traumatically separated from their

parents, caretakers, or other family me
time due to situations such as war and
ger time to overcome such behaviors (

When confronted by traumatic even
regress to an earlier stage of developn
clinging to parents, thumb sucking, sle
a favorite stuffed toy). However, wha
and nurturing exist for a child to regr
raised in the midst of limitless warfare,

Does a child cling to a mother wh
barely able to hold herself up? Do chil
dead father in hopes of receiving his p
realm of the living? What do children l
sessions have been stolen and any pos
existed have faded away? One prized
have is a thumb—a universal comforte
cult to bear.

Emotional Numbing

Survivors of war and terrorism may
astation that is just too severe and unim
tempt to fathom. No words or picture
comes speechless and appears as thou
This ability to mute emotional response
is a means of survival, and it can conti
other life circumstance conjures up the

CULTURAL CONSII

Trauma strikes indiscriminately, re,
cultural background, and the signs of
be universal (Marsella et al., 1996; Kii
of these signs among refugees and im
tance to prevent further suffering and u
and Brook, 1994).

The question is, Can a clinician from
symptoms of a culturally foreign clien

ermeyer, 1985)? The emphasis in Western culture on describing distress psychologically is not shared by every culture. Ethnicity greatly influences what one considers to be a "problem," what one perceives to be the causes of psychological difficulties, and the unique, subjective experience of traumatic stress symptoms (Parson, 1985).

The very idea that PTSD occurs as a normal response to an abnormal situation would suggest that ordinary people can exercise control over their fate—a decidedly optimistic view (McFarlane and Van der Kolk, 1996). Eastern religions, in particular, do not offer the promise to their followers that they will be able to control their destiny. Both Hinduism and Islam teach that life is completely determined by fate and that one has to submit oneself to the will of God or Allah (McFarlane and Van der Kolk, 1996).

The Palestinian community is composed of Muslims, Christians, and Jews. Muslims believe that one should endure life's burdens without complaint, and that only God—not humans—can help people (Awwad, 1999). Christians in the Palestinian community also believe in the will of God, and in fate. Pictures of Jesus Christ, the Virgin Mary, and saints are placed in homes for their protective value and can help maintain a peaceful state of mind (Awwad, 1999).

Samarians in the Palestinian community use a holy artifact called "Joseph's hijab" when a person is suffering from a loss or mental disturbance. Jews also believe that it serves as a remedy and resolves one's difficulties (Awwad, 1999).

Among Arabs, a diagnosis of PTSD has come to be associated with a "noble" and "patriotic" cause, such as the struggle for independence. Strong ties among Arab families appear to shield family members from incidents that otherwise might be experienced as disastrous (Abudabbeh, 1994).

For African peoples, traumatic incidents, such as drought, wars, floods, or epidemics, do not occur by accident or chance. They are usually attributed to God's activity or to a spiritual being (Mbiti, 1990). As a whole, God is not held accountable for such sorrowful events. Instead, "He is brought into the picture primarily as an attempt to explain what is otherwise difficult for the human mind" (Mbiti, 1990, p. 45).

In India, trauma is often viewed as a visitation from malevolent gods. Ideas about astrology and the malevolent influences of the planets on an individual's life are firmly inherent in the Indian psy-

che. Traumas may take place due to th
planets, especially Shani (Saturn). Shri
urn and other planets are located throug

Many Southeast Asians, particularly
that illness is caused by the influenc
Dubrow, and Stamm, 1999). The values
tians, Cambodians, and Vietnamese are
religion (Gerber, Nguyen, and Bounk
that they cannot control their own fate a
of life (Gerber, Nguyen, and Bounkeu:
hill tribe of Laos), symptoms of PTS]
stood within an animist and supernatura
1990).

In many parts of the world personal c
pains and problems (Swartz, 1998). In r
example, psychosomatic complaints (c
stomach upset, dizziness, nerves) are
reported (Gopaul-McNicol and Brice-I

The reason physical complaints are
logical ones is that the majority of peor
conceptualized psychotherapy in the sa
complaints of a physical nature evoke
from others—whereas complaints of a
in a judgment of weakness and failur
(Gopaul-McNicol and Brice-Baker, 19

In Chinese culture, "yin-yang imbala
lation of vital energy (ch'i), and disturba
as well as supernatural powers" are con
problems of a physical nature, which ir
somatic basis for psychological disturba

According to Tseng et al. (1986), er
frustration is not made public or dealt v
for the most part decides on the choice
circumstances, and emphasizes interp
tiveness. A study of depression and P]
gees found that somatization features
because their cultural pattern leans towa
of distress in a somatic idiom. Howeve
aware that their suffering was most like

sadness, anger, losses, and frustrations, as well as to more indigenous explanations, such as spirit loss and spells (Kroll et al., 1989).

For recent migrants coming from areas of considerable social unrest and civil conflict, the diagnosis of PTSD should be considered when the person reports significant somatic and/or psychological distress. Of particular note are symptoms of sleep disturbance and frightening dreams (Friedman, 1997).

SUMMARY

1. Children learn to cope with trauma the best way they know how (via denial, regression, acting out, avoidance, identification with the aggressor, etc.)
2. Post-traumatic stress disorder is the most prevalent and severe type of mental health condition that may follow exposure to a traumatic incident in which there is the presence of real or impending death, serious harm, or risk of grave physical injury to oneself, family, or significant others.
3. PTSD can result from a variety of traumatic incidents, particularly those that involve life threat, and can affect both males and females.
4. PTSD may develop at any age, including childhood.
5. Preschool and school-age children who have been exposed to traumatic incidents often engage in posttraumatic play which involves the reenactment of crucial details of the incident.
6. People who suffer from PTSD continually reexperience the traumatic incident in their minds.
7. Traumatized children remember and relive their experiences not only while awake but also during sleep.
8. Somatic complaints, such as chest pain, stomachaches, and headaches, are frequently reported among traumatized children of all ages.
9. Children who are feeling overwhelmed by direct reminders of the traumatic incident tend to become isolated, find it difficult to concentrate, and can often be seen daydreaming.
10. Traumatized children may experience a sense of hopelessness and pessimism about the future.

11. Following a traumatic incident, cl
    feel guilty for having survived or fc
    tance.
12. Anger may not only reflect the hype
    posttraumatic reactions but also be a
    on by the many disruptions and char
    aftermath of a traumatic incident.
13. Following a traumatic incident, chil
    perience a decline in their school p
14. The effects of trauma, stemming fr
    are usually far more complex, seve
    single-event traumas.
15. The threat of terrorism can persist a
    anxiety and phobic reactions.
16. Long after a terrorist attack or act
    images remain and can awaken me
    form of flashbacks.
17. Trauma strikes indiscriminately, re
    cultural background, and the signs c
    to be universal (Marsella et al., 199
18. The emphasis in Western culture o
    logically is not shared by every cul
19. In many parts of the world personal
    as bodily pains and problems.
20. For recent migrants coming from ar
    rest and civil conflict, the diagnosis
    ered when an individual reports sig
    chological distress. Of particular i
    disturbance and frightening dreams

Chapter 4

Intervention

The persons that arrive have survived which means that they have resources, otherwise they would be dead. A respectful curiosity as to how they managed to survive is a position from which one can learn a lot about their resources, personal, community-bound and cultural/religious/ideological. (Perren-Klinger, 2000, p. 61)

How does one eradicate the experience of a traumatic event or series of ordeals from the life of a child? It is virtually impossible. The child's scars, both emotional and physical, will forever be haunting reminders of uninvited terror.

One can, however, alleviate the pain caused by these scars, whether they are nightmares, flashbacks, anxiety; loss of hope, trust, and autonomy; difficulties with peers; or decline in school performance.

Various modalities have been used in the treatment of traumatized children (e.g., psychodynamic, cognitive-behavioral, and psychopharmacological interventions), including a number of child-related activities (e.g., picture drawing, puppet play, storytelling, and fantasy play).

According to O'Brien (1998), the best general approach in the treatment of PTSD is more likely to be eclectic in nature. Psychotherapy, for example, will be beneficial in engaging traumatized children and preparing them for exposure techniques that will temporarily increase symptomatology. Medication such as selective serotonin reuptake inhibitors (SSRIs) may be helpful to administer, along with psychotherapy.

Kinzie (2001) regards the personality of the therapist, safety, basic trust, decrease in symptomatology, and rebuilding of social relationships, rather than specific treatment techniques, as being the primary needs of those who have been traumatized. The goal of treatment is to

help the child examine, confront, and r
periences and accompanying feelings i
seen on a one-to-one basis, in the cont
situation. Although little empirical su
of individual, group, or family interven
to be most utilized.

The best time to employ trauma-bas
ing the acute phase, when reexperienci
able and the associated affect is most a
1993). "Establishing safety for the ch
pacing disclosure are clinical decisions
and skill" (James, 1994, p. 51).

INDIVIDUAL INTEI

Psychodynamic Therapy

Psychodynamic therapy consists of
more realistic appraisals of his or her a
ways of thinking and coping; a greater s
egies to contain the trauma in tolerable
plying psychodynamic therapy with tra
relative emphasis on the here and now
and deficits that derive from earlier d
shall, Yehuda, and Bone, 2000, p. 351

This intervention is based on unders
conscious meanings that develop withir
aftermath. The approach depends upc
ence. For the younger child, the there
such as dolls representing family memb
or her feelings.

The goals of psychodynamic therap
ber the traumatic events safely; to exp
and feelings associated with those ev
coping skills. The child's family life, p
formance, and emotional and behavi
dressed.

Bob

Bob, a sixteen-year-old boy whose younger brother had drowned in the family swimming pool, began experiencing flashbacks, intrusive thoughts, and recurrent nightmares about the incident. He became socially withdrawn and irritable toward his peers. He avoided swimming pools and a nearby lake where he used to go fishing.

Intervention focused on creating an environment in which Bob could remember his traumatic experience and communicate his associated thoughts and feelings safely. His family life, peer relationships, and emotional and behavioral difficulties were also explored.

During the course of therapy, Bob disclosed that he and his parents had been engaged in a heated argument over his decision not to go to college. They told him that he was a bad influence on his younger brother, Timmy, who had a tendency to mimic his actions. Bob often resented Timmy because he believed Timmy was the "favorite son."

One morning, Bob had just been told by his father what a "loser" he was. Bob responded by going to his room and kicking the wall. He overheard his parents yelling and slamming doors. Moments later, they informed him that they were going out for a while. It was his responsibility to look after Timmy.

Bob decided to hang out by the pool, which was something his younger brother enjoyed. Bob dove into the water and began showing off his swimming techniques. Soon the phone rang. His girlfriend was calling and as they began to converse, he forgot that Timmy was playing by the pool. By the time Bob discovered Timmy's body in the water, it was too late to revive him.

In subsequent sessions, Bob disclosed how he blamed himself for his brother's death, and that once again he had proven himself to be a failure in the eyes of his parents. The focus, therefore, was on helping Bob to express his feelings of sadness, mourn the loss of his brother, and work through his feelings of guilt and shame for not being able to save him.

Counseling the parents allowed them the opportunity to give themselves permission to grieve and to process their feelings of anger. They became aware of their own relationship issues and how their anger was being displaced onto Bob.

Bob's parents were not able to fully resolve their anger, which was in existence before Timmy's drowning, but they were able to see the negative impact it was having on Bob's development as an adolescent and how he had come to view himself.

At some point during the latter phase of therapy, Bob revealed that his parents were separating. He did not appear to be too upset by this news. He ended the session early to go on a fishing excursion with his friends.

Brom, Kleber, and Defares (1989), in a study of the effectiveness of psychotherapeutic methods for the treatment of PTSD, found that psychodynamic therapy was effective in ameliorating trauma-related symptoms, especially those of avoidance. According to Chaffin (2000),

long-term psychodynamic therapy mɛ
younger and less verbal children. It is
dren who are responding to short-term
neously.

Play Therapy

"Play therapy gives the traumatized
through his problems without necessar
own—it belongs to the 'princess' or 'di
'star ship,' not to him" (Terr, 1990, p.
Play therapy can be very useful for tl
or her the opportunity to communicate
ing too much emphasis on verbalization.
storytelling to provide the child opport
of the trauma. The child is able to co
plore fantasies and impulses, and comn
in a safe and nonthreatening environm
The therapist shows these children
repetitive play and their traumatizing
children's dreams, fantasies, and beha
points out the children's defenses. Nev
onstrated to the children during play ar
These traumatized children learn that tt
Several activities and materials are
cluding dolls, puppets, clay, storytellin
that such activities allow children to ɑ
and outcomes and to master feared sit
(Van der Kolk, 1996).

Sheila

Sheila, a six-year-old girl, entered theraр
had been sexually abused by her stepfath
to the session and complained that Sheila
restless during sleep.
It was important to establish a sense of
ship and create a nonthreatening environr
communicate her feelings and concerns. Ir
play (e.g., dolls, puppets, therapeutic boarc

her reenact aspects of her traumatic experience and form a connection between her play and real-life circumstances.

Sheila was apprehensive during her first session without her mother. Efforts were made to reassure her that it was okay and that her mother would remain close by. Sheila was content to hold onto a stuffed panda bear and sit on the child-sized rocking chair in the therapist's office. She seemed intrigued by the display of toys on the shelves and was able to relax a little.

Sheila soon picked up a female doll and engaged in fantasy. She fed the doll and sang a lullaby while the therapist sat and observed. After giving the doll some milk, she put the doll under a blanket and gave her a kiss that involved placing her tongue in the doll's mouth for a period of ten seconds while fondling its vagina. This action was addressed by the therapist and a "feelings chart" was used to help Sheila label her affect. Sheila pointed to the picture of a very sad girl on the feelings chart.

In subsequent sessions, the therapist was invited to actively participate during play. This opportunity was used to model appropriate parent-child interactions and respond to any related concerns. Storytelling was also employed to discuss child abuse, appropriate and inappropriate touching, and other prevention skills.

During the course of therapy, Sheila was able to verbalize her emotions and talk about her stepfather being in jail. At times, she would revert to play or change the subject all together.

Counseling with the mother focused on helping her work through any unresolved issues concerning the sexual abuse of her daughter and the incarceration of her husband. Education of the mother centered on the use of play and storytelling as a means of addressing abuse-related issues with Sheila. The therapist also offered the mother guidance on how to appropriately respond to her daughter's sexually reactive behavior.

Sheila and her mother attended later sessions together to work on their communication skills and learn various coping strategies that would enable them to move on with their lives.

Employing a treatment model for sexually abused preschoolers, Cohen and Mannarino (1993) reported that the therapist might encourage the child to reenact abusive episodes with play materials and consistently model appropriate assertiveness, disclosure, etc. Older children are capable of employing verbal communication in the therapy session. However, it may be easier for some to express trauma-related feelings and relay their experiences through role-play, games, puppets, or drawing pictures (Brooks and Siegel, 1996).

Cognitive-Behavioral Therapy

The goal of cognitive-behavioral therapy (CBT) is to help the traumatized child make sense of what happened and to help him or her

master feelings of anxiety and helpless
1999). The type of format that a clinic
termined by the nature of the traumati
accident, homicide). The child is taug
anxiety (with deep-breathing exercises,
and negative thoughts, as well as ange

It is important to normalize reactio
child reintegrate and restructure cognit
cific problems in the areas of family ai
management will need to be addressed
Empirical data appear to strongly sup
other forms of psychotherapy in allev
children. CBT, for example, has been s
sexually abused children.

- In a treatment outcome study for
  Cohen and Mannarino (1993) fou
  inappropriate behaviors respond
  interventions than to play therapy
- Deblinger, McLeer, and Henry (1
  tion of cognitive-behavioral pare
  effectively ameliorate PTSD in so
  on findings in their study of this
  teen.
- March, Amaya-Jackson, and Mu
  improvement in children and ado
  treated with CBT. No relapse was
  continued.

The major behavioral methods utili:
uals diagnosed with PTSD include the
stress inoculation, and systematic des
techniques may be applied to traumat

Exposure Therapy

Exposure therapy involves the syst
fears (e.g., trauma-associated thoughts
of the traumatic event, such as the loca
ows and Foa, 2000). The methods of e

frontation with frightening, yet realistically safe, stimuli that continues until anxiety is reduced" (Rothbaum and Schwartz, 2002, p. 59).

"Exposure gradually alters behavior, physiology, and cognitions by habituation" (Marks et al., 1998, p. 322) and has been found to be effective in the reduction of PTSD symptoms (Tarrier et al., 1999; Marks et al., 1998). This approach may be less appropriate, however, with children who have acting-out behaviors, are not symptomatic, or are showing spontaneous improvement (Chaffin, 2000).

Eye movement desensitization reprocessing (EMDR) is a recently developed method of individual psychotherapy that involves the integration of exposure and client-centered principles (Greenwald, 1999). The standard EMDR protocol (Shapiro, 1989) is reviewed by Greenwald (1999), who applies a similar procedure in his work with older children and adolescents:

- *Imagery*—The client is instructed to select an image that represents the key moment from the memory, possibly the most distressing or intrusive image.
- *Negative cognition*—The client is instructed to describe the negative belief about the self that emerges from the memory.
- *Positive cognition*—The client is instructed to select a more positive, adaptive belief about the self, even if it does not feel entirely accurate before reprocessing.
- *Validity of Cognition (VoC) Scale*—The client is asked to rate the positive cognition on a scale from one to seven, with one being completely false and seven being completely true.
- *Emotion*—The client is instructed to describe his or her current emotional response to the selected memory image.
- *Subjective Units of Disturbance Scale (SUDS)*—The client is asked to rate the current intensity of the negative emotion on a scale from zero to ten, with zero being no disturbance and ten being the most intense disturbance imaginable.
- *Physical sensation*—The client is instructed to report the location of any physical sensation that may accompany his or her current response to this concentration on the traumatic memory.
- *Eye movements*—Rapid bilateral eye movements are utilized to promote the accessing, reprocessing, and integration of the target memory. The therapist induces eye movements by having the client visually track the therapist's moving fingers (or some

other item, such as a pen or poi
plished at the pace of approximate
per second, twenty to thirty times,
from the client's face. The rate,
ments, and interim may vary. The
with focus on the targeted memo
the different aspects of the memo
This is called the desensitization
tive cognition is "installed" by foc
ments (installation phase of treatn
the target memory and the positive
or her body for any tension or dis
gering (body scan phase of treatn
client to relax again before leaving
treatment). At the start of each sess
of EMDR, a reevaluation is perfc
treatment and to determine the ne>

Greenwald (1999) modifies the standa
younger children by reducing the dura
and increasing the amount of parental i

Exposure therapies can take the form
exposure. Imaginal exposure (flooding)
feared events or memories of the traum
In vivo exposure involves the child ren
the actual stimuli (Bryant and Harvey, 2

According to Saigh, Yule, and Inamd
have difficulty imagining traumatic ma
laxation procedures, or tolerating prolor
suggest that, under these circumstance
have the children make drawings of the
verbally describe them rather than subj

When the length of exposure to a
termed *implosive therapy* (Joseph, Wil
cording to Bryant and Harvey (2000), it
find it difficult to comprehend the ration
traumatized by focusing on the traumati
ods; and may be unable to employ cogn
beliefs about the imagery. It is therefo
used in applying implosive therapy to c

Occasionally, when a child is undergoing exposure treatment, the degree of affective response may be too much for him or her to manage. When there is difficulty moderating this affective arousal in the session, anxiety management techniques may be introduced. The aim of this approach is to offer clients enough control to remain exposed to the anxiety-provoking stimuli, until they undergo some amount of habituation (Richards and Lovell, 1999). Although it is necessary for exposure therapy to be sufficiently long, repetitive, and detailed, it is important to go at the client's own pace (Rothbaum and Schwartz, 2002).

Mark

Mark, a seventeen-year-old boy, was swimming at the beach when he was attacked by a shark. A portion of his right leg was severed as he tried to escape. Mark never returned to the beach and became fearful of swimming activities, avoiding them entirely. He experienced nightmares and a decline in his schoolwork.

Mark's parents brought him to therapy. Initially, the focus of intervention was the establishment of a therapeutic relationship and sense of trust. Mark was then instructed on the use of relaxation techniques and positive self-talk. During the course of therapy, he began to show some improvement in his school performance. It took several months for Mark to master the techniques, however. Once this task was accomplished, he was ready for the next phase of treatment: exposure therapy.

Mark returned to the beach, accompanied by the therapist. He was asked to recall his traumatic experience while remaining as relaxed as possible. The therapist raised various questions, such as, "What are you doing at this moment? What do you see? What are you hearing? What is your reaction? What are you feeling?" in attempts to re-create the incident.

The therapist calmly coached Mark while he was being exposed to anxiety-generating cues. For example, the therapist said, "Imagine you are at the beach during spring break. Allow yourself to revisit the waters where the shark attacked you. What do you see? What is happening?"

While the scene of the trauma was being devised, the therapist started out with low doses of anxiety-generating cues and gradually moved up to higher doses, along with instructions on the use of relaxation techniques. Mark's negative trauma associations were eventually deconditioned and replaced with more positive ones. He was encouraged to hold onto his gains by resuming the swimming activities that he once feared. The therapist also encouraged Mark to utilize the coping strategies that he learned in his sessions to aid him in confronting trauma-related memories and stimuli.

Stress Inoculation Training (SIT)

Stress inoculation training (SIT) is t
ety management. It involves techniqu
ation skills, guided self-talk, role-play
control, and covert modeling (Peterso

Foa et al. (1991), in their study of
victims, found that SIT was the most
prolonged exposure appeared to be t
term. According to Pynoos and Nader
are often recommended for adults and
lowing a traumatic event and may acut
relief from anxiety.

Lisa

Lisa, a six-year-old female, was playing
ground when a man fired a gun from a m
tended target and shot Lisa's friend instea
her friend's blood splattered onto the pave
She became hysterical and had to be car
ambulance arrived. Lisa's friend died on th

Since the tragic incident, Lisa was afra
men" hiding in the bushes and plotting to
was going to kill the bad men and make h

By the time Lisa entered therapy, she wa
to school, insomnia, intrusions, and hyper
during the course of therapy included biofe
management (e.g., progressive muscle re
scription of clonidine was also utilized to
hypervigilance, and insomnia.

Lisa was made aware of her maladapti
the bad men would come after her and sh
She was instructed on the use of positive s
ever a negative thought attempted to intrud
used to practice positive strategies for cop
These behavioral interventions and the ad
Lisa establish increased control over her t

Systematic Desensitization

When the duration of exposure is bri
low, it is termed *systematic desensiti*

Yule, 1997). In systematic desensitization, the child's fear is deconditioned. In other words, the child, who is accompanied by the therapist, undergoes gradual exposure to less-feared objects, while being shown simultaneously how to relax until he or she is able to face the most feared object successfully (Monahon, 1993).

According to Gaensbauer and Siegel (1995), desensitization procedures in the early months of infancy will probably involve direct interaction between the caregiver and infant around the crucial caregiving routines that have been disrupted (e.g., feeding and sleeping).

Parson (1997, p. 188) applied play desensitization techniques to children exposed to community violence; specific toys and other play materials were arranged in configurations that "distally and proximally resemble the original traumatic situation." A hierarchical order was used consisting of low-anxiety to high-anxiety cues.

Carla

Carla, a three-year-old girl, entered therapy following a house fire that left her family homeless. The fire occurred in the evening, while she, her two older siblings, and their father were sleeping. Carla's mother was tired from working extra hours at the hospital and decided to curl up on the couch and smoke a cigarette. She tossed the cigarette into the wastebasket, unaware that it was still lit. She then went up to her room and fell asleep.

Carla and the rest of her family awakened to the blaring of the smoke alarm. The hallway and their rooms were filled with smoke. Fire appeared to be consuming everything in sight as Carla's father carried her out the window to some neighbors standing outside. The firemen rushed to rescue the rest of Carla's family. Fortunately, no casualties occurred, but the whole family had to be transported by ambulance to a nearby hospital where they were treated for smoke inhalation.

Carla's parents expressed concern when she began manifesting symptoms of increased anxiety, avoidance of her mother, and clinginess toward her father. She was easily startled and hypersensitive to loud sounds, the sight of fire, and the smell of smoke. She refused to sleep alone and became afraid of the dark.

During the therapy session with her parents, Carla initially reenacted various aspects of her traumatic experience using toy cars, trucks, a dollhouse, and doll figures representing herself, family members, and firefighters. She responded by putting a girl doll in the bedroom and placing it under her bed. As Carla became comfortable with the playroom, the therapist placed the girl doll on the bed instead of under it and three other dolls in separate bedrooms. The mother doll was situated downstairs on the couch.

The therapist then demonstrated the
cigarette in a wastebasket as the mother
angry expression on her face and walked
excessively tight. She stomped her feet se
turning to the activity.

The therapist removed the doll figures f
the hallway, while making coughing soun
what the therapist was trying to demonstra
jumped into her father's lap and pushed
knowledge her mother's attempts to offer
establish a connection between the reena
tional and behavioral responses. The ther
fearfulness, anger, and need to feel safe.

Carla appeared to be relieved by the the
She approached the fire scene activity aga
vited to participate. The therapist arrange
out in sequential order similar to the actua
coughing and choking vigorously. Her fa
Carla by using his doll figure to help lift t
house and into the arms of other doll figu
noises, pretending that the fire trucks and
rescue and bringing them to the hospital.

The therapist enlisted the mother's par
ing the girl doll at the hospital. At that mor
the doll away from her mother and shoutin
to cry. Her mother, who was also crying, a
had not noticed that the cigarette was still
replied, "But you're the mommy! You did
mother were able to help Carla understanc
mies, can make mistakes, and how impor
takes so no one gets hurt again.

As the mother's comfort level improved
play materials at home in order to reconn
munication between them. Fire safety liter
Carla and her family feel secure again and
tool.

Desensitization techniques were emplo
the dark and sleeping alone. These incluc
while in the company of family, sleeping in
sleeping by herself first with the light on,
flashlight, and the light off.

Further application of play therapy an
sulted in a reduction of Carla's trauma-relat
with a safe environment in which to relive h
cess her associated feelings, she was able
and the level of communication between th

Drell, Siegel, and Gaensbauer (1993) describe an interactionally based behavioral desensitization program that can be used to help infants re-create and assimilate their traumatic experiences:

- The infants are exposed to anxiety-provoking cues and/or situations in small, graduated doses in closer and closer approximation to whatever the adverse situation and related cues may be (e.g., being fed, sitting in a high chair, or being touched).
- For infants under six months of age, desensitization techniques give emphasis to concrete interactional encounters that involve the actual distress situation, with the caregiver or therapist as the main stimulus.
- In the latter half of the first year, the desensitization techniques used to reconstruct the trauma refer more precisely to those elements or situations that are trauma related, aside from the interactive elements.
- By the second year, traumatic experiences tend to be reenacted through play materials and sensorimotor activity.
- By the latter half of the second year, verbal communication is used to aid in interpretation (e.g., the labeling of emotions).

Larry

Larry, a seven-month-old boy, was abused and neglected by his grandfather. The grandfather hit Larry in the face several times, urinated on him, and locked him up in a dark closet by himself while hammering his fist on the door from the outside.

This abuse was repeated for several weeks until Larry's mother returned home early from work one day. She wanted to surprise Larry with a new train set that she had purchased for his birthday. To her horror, she discovered Larry screaming in the closet, red in the face, and trembling, as he lay on the floor reeking of urine. His grandfather was in the bathroom taking a shower.

At the time of therapy, Larry was exhibiting posttraumatic symptoms— increased levels of hyperarousal, sleep disturbances, fearfulness, excessive crying, and resistance to touch. Intervention involved the use of comforting techniques (e.g., holding, infant massage, swaddling, rocking) and other calming stimuli (e.g., cuddly toys, soft tones, soothing music, warm baths, and gentle facial expressions). Larry's parents were instructed in the use of these techniques and applied them at home for several weeks, despite resistance. Larry began to show signs of calming down in response to his mother holding him close and whispering into his ear. He even produced an occasional smile and his anxiety level was subsequently reduced.

GROUP INTERVE

Children are seen together in a grou
the opportunity to disclose and discus
tions to traumatic incidents in an atmc
sive. The assumption is that this type of
the recovery and adjustment process (C

Group therapy is often used when 1
exposed to a common traumatic incide
be optimal for situations of this nature. '
children in processing any feelings of f
lated to the traumatic incident. Psychoec
symptoms is also provided.

The goal of therapy is for group mer
standing of all the elements of their trau
a sense of trust and confidence. If a chil
ual counseling, group therapy can serv
Group therapy may also be used as a pr
be less suitable for children with avoi
pression (Chaffin, 2000).

Advantages of Group Therapy

- Group therapy alleviates the lonel
  hon, 1993).
- Group therapy provides member
  and support (Scurfield, 1985).
- When sitting with a group of pee
  traumatic experiences, members n
  that something is wrong with ther
- Group therapy offers members the
  their feelings and to work throug
  lated to the trauma (Scurfield, 198

Chard, Resick, and Wertz (1999) des
cessing therapy in group work with
session group is conducted in weekly n
ably with coleaders.

Session 1: Introduction and Education Phase

- The therapist (group leader) provides information about the development of PTSD and outlines the course of treatment.
- For homework, each group member is to write about what it means to have been raped in connection to the following elements: safety, trust, power, control, esteem, and intimacy.

Session 2: Meaning of the Event

- The group members review their previously assigned homework and share their reactions.
- "Stuck points" are identified. The leader then facilitates the discussion of four basic emotional reactions (mad, sad, glad, and scared) and helps increase the group's understanding of the relationship between their thoughts and feelings.
- Related homework is assigned.

Session 3: Identification of Thoughts and Feelings

- Homework is reviewed and stuck points are identified.
- Group members are assigned additional homework which entails writing a detailed account of the rape, including as many sensory details (sights, sounds, smells, etc.), thoughts, and feelings that they can recall. They are instructed to read it at least once before their next session.

Session 4: Remembering the Rape

- The leader subjects each member to details of the rape that have been avoided to allow the member's emotions to be expressed and extinguished.
- Previously assigned homework is discussed. Additional homework entails writing the entire account of the rape again, adding more sensory details, thoughts, and feelings. The account is to be read daily prior to the next session.

Session 5: Identification of Stuck Point

- Members discuss their reactions t
  work. Differences and similarities
  time of the rape and how they felt
  addressed.
- For homework, each member cho
  answers challenging questions in

Session 6: Challenging Questions

- Members share their homework re
  the leader, analyze and confront th
- For homework, members discuss
  previous ones, and how they fit wi

Session 7: Faulty Thinking Patterns

- Patterns are discussed in terms of
  and can lead to negative feelings a
- Homework for sessions 7 to 11 invo

Session 8: Safety Issues

- Members review homework, focu
  about safety can elicit anxiety and
  ior.

Session 9: Trust Issues

- Members review homework, focus

Session 10: Power and Control Issues

- Leaders help members to strike
  complete control versus feeling co
- Members are asked to practice g
  ments and to do, unconditionally
  themselves every day.

Session 11: Esteem Issues

- Members discuss previously assigned homework.
- The leader helps members realize that bad things can happen to good people.
- For additional homework, members are to rewrite their first assignment on what it means to have been raped.

Session 12: Intimacy Issues and Meaning of the Event

- Members review previously assigned homework to identify stuck points and to change cognitions in order to enhance intimacy.
- Members discuss their reactions to the homework and compare them to their reactions to the same homework when it was first assigned.
- Members are encouraged to look at how their beliefs have changed and to identify faulty thinking that may need additional intervention.
- Skills and progress are reviewed.

Debriefings

Debriefings are formal group meetings that are usually led by mental health professionals. Debriefings have been applied to various groups besides emergency workers, such as school communities, corporations, neighborhoods, etc. The meetings offer survivors opportunities to discuss their traumatic experiences and develop more realistic and accurate appraisals of what happened. The survivors are able to share with others who have gone through similar experiences and learn that they are not alone and are not "going insane."

Debriefings also have an educational component that involves teaching the survivors about the signs of stress and various coping strategies available and offering referral information. There is a seven-phase structure (Mitchell and Dyregrov, 1993) involved whereby ground rules are introduced; survivors report the facts of what happened; describe their thoughts about it; discuss their emotions regarding their traumatic experience; review their signs of stress; learn coping strategies; and are given opportunity for closure.

Following is a debriefing format c
(O'Brien, 1998; Mitchell and Dyregro
terbury and Yule, 1999):

Introduction

- Introduce the debriefing team an
- Provide participants with inforn
  ground, why you are here, and th
- Explain the purpose of the debrie
- Discuss guidelines concerning n
  using mobile phones/pagers, talk
  judging others, protecting confid
  group.

The Facts

- Ask each participant to describe i
  of involvement in the traumatic in
  about what happened, beginning
- Ask for any sensations (e.g., sigh
  may have experienced during the

Thoughts About the Incident

- Ask participants to share what
  their minds during and after the i

Reactions to the Incident

- Ask participants to share any en
  they had during and after the inci

Education

- Educate participants concerning
  that might result from the incider
- Normalize signs of distress, and
  manage them.

- Provide helpful handouts to aid in their recovery (e.g., dealing with grief and loss; anger management; suggestions on how to cope following a traumatic incident; common responses to trauma; and guidelines for families and friends of survivors).

Closure

- Provide a summary of the meeting.
- Acknowledge that a speedy recovery could still be followed by serious symptoms. Offer participants referral sources within their local community, should their distress persist for too long or recur.

A School Shooting

Michael, a fifteen-year-old boy, was recently suspended from school. He showed up in the cafeteria dressed in black with a vacant look on his face. He jumped onto a table, pulled out a gun, and shot his math teacher, Ms. Henderson, at close range. The students and staff responded with shock, fear, and panic. They raced toward the nearest exit as Michael fired shots at random. Many people were hit and fell to the ground, their blood splattering the floor.

The school principal and a teacher were able to restrain Michael until the police arrived. Michael was taken into custody, and the school was evacuated. The students were terrified and trembling as they were reunited with their parents. News cameras moved quickly on the scene to "zoom in" on their pain. The school staff and faculty gathered together but were quite numb from the experience. It was a nightmare everyone wanted to wake up from. Unfortunately, six students and one teacher wouldn't wake up from this horror. They lost their lives.

Three days after the incident, a debriefing team was called to the school to offer services to faculty and staff. Community agencies, grief counselors, and the teaching staff were already assisting the students individually, in small groups, and in the classroom as needed.

The school principal arranged for all faculty and staff to participate in the debriefing when school was not in session. The participants were introduced to the debriefing facilitator and cofacilitator, who explained the purpose of the debriefing, proposed benefits, and guidelines. Each participant then took turns describing, in order of occurrence, the facts about what happened during the day of the shooting and their level of involvement. Following is a description of a debriefing exercise.

PARTICIPANT A: I was on cafeteria duty assisting with food preparation and cleanup. I remember looking up and seeing the boy with a gun. It was like something straight out of a movie. He just shot Ms. Henderson—one of

the teachers—directly in the head. I co
horrifying.

PARTICIPANT B: I'm the school nurse. It was
dents and staff until the ambulances a
chaos. I tried my best to stop the bleed
another in the arm, and Mr. Smith was
child didn't get shot, but hurt her leg in t
trying to escape.

FACILITATOR: Did you experience any partic
you remember hearing a particular sou
out in your memory?

PARTICIPANT C: The gunshots. I was sitting
ing a sandwich, when all of a sudden I h
screaming. Once I realized what was
dents out of there. It was like I was mov
rang through my ears. I couldn't believe

PARTICIPANT A: There was so much blood o
Henderson. I didn't see anyone else ge
kitchen. I just wanted the nightmare to

FACILITATOR: What thoughts did you have

PARTICIPANT D: I was thinking of the safety c
just pumping as I ushered them through
well. I was apprehensive all the while,
would be more snipers hiding in the bu

PARTICIPANT E: I was trying to plot a way to
class and I figured maybe I could get ins
what made him tick. My plan was to ca
gun, like federal agents do in hostage
mapped out in my head, but I couldn't r

FACILITATOR: What thoughts have you had

PARTICIPANT F: I found myself questioning
working in this community. There has b
rounding neighborhoods. That's all you
time was different. Ms. Henderson was
was a very dear friend. Those six stude
my own children. I loved each of them
tears.] My heart goes out to their familie
ing.

FACILITATOR: What were your reactions du

PARTICIPANT G: I felt nauseous—like I was
that pool of blood on the floor. It was sc
want to think about it anymore or I'm lia

PARTICIPANT B: I couldn't feel anything. It w

PARTICIPANT D: I remember my palms being sweaty and feeling so anxious. My heart was racing a mile a minute. I just told myself that the nightmare would soon be over.

FACILITATOR: Has anyone experienced difficulty sleeping since the incident?

PARTICIPANT A: I haven't been able to sleep through the night since witnessing Ms. Henderson get shot in the head. It was so gory. I have nightmares about it.

PARTICIPANT B: I keep hearing the sounds of gunshots every time I try to sleep. Any loud noise reminds me of it—*Bang! Bang!*

FACILITATOR: What other reactions have you experienced since the incident?

PARTICIPANT D: I haven't been out with my friends since the shooting. I'm afraid some gangster is going to attack me or something. It just isn't safe anymore. I won't even let my children go to the park and play. They can get hurt or shot at, for no reason at all.

PARTICIPANT E: I've been feeling extremely guilty for not taking action when I had the chance. Those children did not have to die. I should have done something to save them instead of standing there like a scared rabbit.

FACILITATOR: What you all have described are normal reactions to a rather abnormal situation. You are not going insane. It's not every day that a person just walks into a school and shoots at everyone in sight, so of course some of you are going to feel anxious, numb, nauseous, and insecure. Those are just a few of the signs associated with what is called posttraumatic stress. Anyone who has been involved in a traumatic incident will experience some form of posttraumatic stress. As a result, you may undergo a variety of emotional, behavioral, and physical reactions associated with that incident. Many of you have described feeling guilty, fearful, helpless, and unsafe. Others have mentioned having difficulty sleeping and socializing with friends. You may also have reminders of the incident that are likely to trigger painful emotions and thoughts associated with your experience. The sounds of gunshots, the sight of blood, and loud screams are just some of the triggers that were mentioned by the group. There are various ways you can take care of yourselves and cope with what has happened. You can reach out to family and friends who care about you or join a support group. It is important not to be alone at a time like this, and rely on the support and strength of others. It is also helpful to stick to your usual routine. Keep your life running the way it was prior to the incident. It is not a good idea to make life-changing decisions right now, such as quitting your profession and moving to a small town in Kansas. Your adrenaline is high. Several thoughts may be racing through your head. It would be difficult to make major decisions—decisions that you are likely to regret later on—at this juncture, so slow down. It would be beneficial to participate in activities that are healthy, relaxing, positive, and enjoyable to you, such as exercise, deep-breathing techniques, meditation, listening to music, singing, and socializing with friends, even when you don't feel like it. These coping strategies tend to help alleviate trauma-related stress, and promote a positive well-being. This is a time when

you're most vulnerable, so avoid negativ
hol or drugs, overeating, gambling, uns
activities will only make matters worse. If
havioral, and physical reactions to the
and debilitating, you may wish to conside
ful at any time. My cofacilitator will be giv
you information on posttraumatic stress
ing strategies, and community resources
beneficial to you. We want to thank you
you to partake of some nourishing snack
in the lobby. Please feel free to ask us an
leaving.

Debriefing has been used in various
is strongly supported. However, there is
ficacy as a preventive intervention in te
ity (O'Brien, 1998). Debriefing is not t
sult in negative effects. Caution must
techniques, and sufficient training is es
1999; O'Brien, 1998).

FAMILY INTERVI

The entire family is affected when a
posed to a traumatic incident and suffers
ily therapy may involve all of the mem
Families experience a range of em
frustration, alienation, hurt, shame, anc
is easily irritated, loses interest in family
bers of the family, becomes reckless, or
Family members may feel that they h
no one understands what they are goin
apy setting, the therapist observes how
with one another and offers empathy, su
to cope more effectively. According to
is not only a method of treatment but a
alternative means of observing, prevel
disorders.
The goals for family therapy to aid th
child's affective responses instead of (

the child a sense of personal security; and helping the family to allevi-ate secondary stresses and adversities (Pynoos and Nader, 1993).

PHARMACOLOGICAL INTERVENTIONS

Pharmacotherapy is rarely the treatment of choice during an acute phase of trauma. More often, it is recommended as an adjunctive form of symptom relief, primarily to help the child become more re-ceptive to and more capable of participating in other forms of treat-ment (Arroyo and Eth, 1996).

Donnelly and Amaya-Jackson (2002) recommend the following sequential steps in selecting medication for the treatment of PTSD:

- Obtain an accurate diagnosis.
- Identify the presence of any comorbid conditions (e.g., attach-ment disorder, attention-deficit hyperactivity disorder [ADHD], or depression).
- Identify target symptoms for intervention and specify reason-able treatment objectives.
- Determine the appropriate intervention (e.g., cognitive-behav-ioral therapy versus pharmacological treatment).

Davidson and Van der Kolk (1996) mention the following princi-pal goals for using medications in PTSD:

- Reduction in symptoms of intrusion and avoidance
- Reduction in symptoms of hyperarousal
- Improvement in symptoms of depression and numbing
- Reduction in overinterpreting incoming stimuli as reminders of the trauma
- Reduction in symptoms of dissociation and psychoses
- Reduction in symptoms of aggression to self and others

Medication can help older children reduce symptoms such as the anxiety, depression, and insomnia associated with PTSD. Children with symptoms of hyperarousal (intense fear, anxiety, anger, and panic, in response to even minor stimuli) are vulnerable to sleep prob-lems, both because they cannot console themselves enough to go to

sleep and because they may be afraid o
(Davidson and Van der Kolk, 1996).

According to Davidson and Van der
best treated with any of the drugs that rec
as benzodiazepines or clonidine. Cloni
in reducing symptoms of aggression, h
culties in a sample of preschoolers witl
Riggs, 1996). Benzodiazepines have be
tioned and generalized arousal in anima
Van der Kolk, 1996).

SSRIs tend to be the medication of ch
dren due to their minimal side effects,
ports their efficacy in the treatment of ar
Kolk (1996) reported that once an indiv
clinician should first choose either an S
sant, and expect to introduce a second d
a mood stabilizer, or a benzodiazepine)
only a partial response.

In their study of adolescent friends c
colleagues (1995) reported that due to tl
anxiety, depression, and PTSD, treatme
help alleviate symptoms in those sufferi

The appropriateness of the use of n
toddlers is not fully determined at prese
The empirical data that examine the us
with PTSD, in general, have been quite
approaches should be given first conside
unless such approaches have not been su
tion and/or the continuation of sympto
ability to function.

SCHOOL-BASED INTE

Interventions may work best in sch
comfortable, and natural environment tl
therapy in the school setting, for examp
ise as a preventive mode for handling l
have undergone similar terrors.

The following principles, according to Williams (1994), are considered paramount to counseling traumatized children in a school setting:

- Establish a safe environment for the child.
- Expect to be tested by the child over a long period of time.
- Show empathy.
- Teach the child about the nature of grief, as well as normal stress and posttraumatic stress reactions.
- Help the child work through his or her memories of the trauma.
- Help the child identify and express his or her feelings.
- Help the child acknowledge and deal with losses that have resulted from the trauma.
- Help the child establish appropriate peer and other relationships.
- Establish a treatment plan.
- Become familiar with various treatment models
- Help empower the child.

The broad use of school-based interventions (classroom, individual, and group therapy) was supported in a study by Goenjian et al. (1997). Children feel supported when they hear their peers discussing their own traumatic experiences. Their emotional and behavioral reactions are validated and normalized.

Schools are developing counseling programs for students and maintaining a referral base of counseling professionals within their community. Some schools even have social workers and/or psychologists on staff to attend to the counseling needs of students and provide on-site consultation to school personnel. Guidance counselors are also available to students in need of supportive counseling.

Examples of some school-based interventions include curricula that address traumatic incidents and signs of stress; group activities and discussion; and coping strategies such as painting, drawing, storytelling, and play (Pfefferbaum, 1997). Pynoos and Nader (1993) caution against the use of classroom interventions as a substitute for individual and family interventions.

The following sections list suggested activities to help children following a traumatic incident.

Children's Activities

1. Invite the children to draw picture
each take turns describing their drawin;
drawings make them feel. Explain that
ings and not to keep them all bottled u
ture of what it feels like to keep all thei
all of their drawings into a bottle). Let t¹
listen and that you care. They will fee
you, their parents, friends, and others ¹

2. Practice deep-breathing exercise;
student take five deep breaths, slowly e
plain how soothing and relaxing this ⁴
afraid or worried. Provide the follow
balloon until it pops in the air. Explain ¹
all our feelings inside and do not talk a¹
just going to burst. Blow up another b₂
pop, slowly release the air out of it. E>
share their feelings with others, they s¹
they may feel in doing the deep-breath¹

3. Involve the class in storytelling. S
overcame a difficult time and had a ha¹

4. Have the class participate in a ph}
ball, exercising, or dancing. Explain ho¹
feel better.

5. Have the class do something wit¹
clay figures or finger painting.

6. Play music and sing songs out lou
help alleviate stress.

7. Invite the students to construct a
who was hospitalized.

8. Have toys available (e.g., soft cud¹
tion toys to help relieve anxiety, and ꞓ
express feelings). Encourage positive ²

Activities for Adolescents

1. Encourage students to record the³
   the incident in a journal.
2. Invite the students to design a get-
   dent or faculty member.

3. Have the students design a yearbook page for the deceased.
4. Encourage students to write down or record anything they would have wanted to tell the deceased if given the opportunity.
5. Have the students express their feelings about the incident with artwork or poetry writing.
6. Brainstorm positive ways to cope with the traumatic incident.
7. Invite the students to gather notes of encouragement to send to the family of the deceased.
8. Prepare for attendance at memorial or funeral service.
9. Provide opportunity for physical exercise.
10. Ask the students to compose a song about their experience and feelings.

CULTURAL CONSIDERATIONS

"Culture is a remarkable human invention not only because it allows us to adapt and survive, but also because it requires us to make meaning of the world and our lives" (Podolefsky and Brown, 1997, p. 9).

As cultural and ethnic diversities increase in the United States, so does the need to offer specific modes of therapy to diverse clients (Tanaka-Matsumi, Seiden, and Lam, 2001). Return to the home country for psychiatric care may not be desirable or even feasible (Westermeyer, 1985). This presents a unique challenge to caregivers that seek to practice effectively in the new millennium. Caregivers will be called on more and more to treat immigrant children who may differ not only in language but also in culture or worldview.

To provide culturally sensitive treatment to ethnic minority children and adolescents, Porter (2000) recommends that therapists be cognizant of acculturation issues, stereotypes, different modes of communication (verbal and nonverbal), sociocultural conditions, ethnic minority identity development, and the impact of racism and oppression on the psychological development of ethnic minority youth.

The history and current status of one's ethnic group in society, personal encounters with prejudice, and one's reaction to awareness of stereotypes and prejudice are some of the factors likely to coincide in affecting psychological outcomes (Phinney, 1996). The issues of

transference and countertransference
treatment process of ethnic minority y

> If psychodynamic processes shou
> of our ancestors—into the life ex
> ones; into the days of slavery,
> sion—what emotions do these no
> someone whom we feel (in our fa
> pressive role in that historical pa
> tory transmitted to us by each gen
> reminded by society that we may
> part of conquered nations or imp
> the constant reminder that someo
> psyche? It is impossible to detern
> the painful past forms part of our
> react in a healing relationship
> sciously we associate with that p
> 2000, p. 20)

According to Peddle et al. (1999), a
social area, whether during situations
work holistically with people in the cc
culture. Trauma can be understood o
ideological systems and spiritual pract

When cultural meanings are translat
son or applied universally, it is usuall
Until recently, most training institutior
fessionals to employ the etic approach
ment of culturally diverse clients. Ac
Soriano (2000), this approach does n
cultures; it focuses on common theme
and psychotherapy. The term *emic,* on
tural meanings that are derived from i
assumed to be specific to that culture (

According to Cuéllar and Paniagua
mental health professionals to discove
to commence a professional expeditio
fellow human and cultural beings. Ho
cians to move from a universal approac
that acknowledges the client's unique

and Paniagua, 2000). Culture-specific treatment should be offered to ethnically diverse clients, particularly to those who are unacculturated or who possess very traditional ethnic values which are discrepant from Western values (Kurasaki et al., 2000).

Much debate is based on whether the treatment of posttraumatic stress symptoms can be applied universally. According to Marsella et al. (1996), it appears that trauma-based interventions may be applicable to non-Western individuals with PTSD. Behavior therapy, for example, is practiced in many areas where the indigenous sociocultural background is quite different from the Caucasian culture in which it originated (De Silva and Samarasinghe, 1985). Behavioral techniques apparently work well regardless of the patient's literacy, education, or cultural beliefs. Cognitive therapies can also be applied without necessarily knowing a great amount about the patient's culture.

Western therapeutic approaches proved to be effective in the treatment of posttraumatic stress symptoms of adolescents who had been exposed to an earthquake in Armenia (Goenjian et al., 1997). When clonidine was included in the treatment of Southeast Asian refugees diagnosed with PTSD, they reported a decrease in nightmares, irritability, and startle responses (Kinzie et al., 1990). Debriefings are other methods of intervention that have been applied to various cultures and countries following traumatic incidents (Dyregrov, 1997). Chemtob et al. (1997) assessed two groups of survivors who had been debriefed following their exposure to Hurricane Iniki in Hawaii. They found that the debriefing intervention contributed to a significant decrease in hurricane-related distress.

The following sections discuss some of the factors involving the use of individual, family, and group therapy with diverse cultures.

Individual Therapy

- The disadvantage to seeing some clients on a one-to-one basis is when they come from cultures (such as most non-Westernized societies) in which one's sense of individuality and autonomy is either discouraged or not considered to be of primary importance (Gopaul-McNicol and Brice-Baker, 1998).
- The advantage to seeing some clients on a one-to-one basis is that they receive needed assistance without having to face family disap-

proval due to the stigma associated v
quest of psychological services (
Baker, 1998).

Family Therapy

* Family therapy is a good modality fc
  cultures where the needs and goals o
  the needs and goals of the individual
  Baker, 1998).
* An advantage of family therapy is
  viewpoint that does not search for ill
  dividuals. This is especially importa
  therapy is a negative choice (Gopa
  1998).
* It is important that family therapy ap
  tributes of the extended family syste
  extended family in the therapy proce
  ethnic minority groups to work in an
  represents their real-life experience
  facilitates the therapeutic process an
  ing (Wilson, Kohn, and Lee, 2000).
* Expanding treatment beyond the im
  the likelihood that support and progr
  therapy will continue after terminat
  2000).

Group Therapy

* The main task in providing group the
  "promote trust and safety within th
  lives" (Han and Vasquez, 2000, p. 1
* In homogeneous groups, members l
  characteristics in common (Han and
* Groups that are topic specific for a pa
  likely to be successful when the gro
  McNicol and Brice-Baker, 1998).
* An advantage of having homogeneit
  ease in sharing unique cultural exper
  of questions pertaining to identity (I

- A disadvantage of homogeneous groups is that the leaders and members may assume similarities and de-emphasize differences (Han and Vasquez, 2000).
- Heterogeneous groups are made up of members from both the majority culture and subcultures in the United States (Han and Vasquez, 2000).
- A disadvantage of heterogeneous groups is the sense of being "the only one." This experience can be isolating and make it difficult for that member to relate to others in the group (Han and Vasquez, 2000).
- If the group is heterogeneous, more than two ethnic minorities should be present to avoid the probability of anyone being scapegoated (Gopaul-McNicol and Brice-Baker, 1998).
- It is important to be mindful of language when providing group therapy. Asians, for example, are quite diverse. Putting them all in the same group ignores the language barrier (Gopaul-McNicol and Brice-Baker, 1998).
- Group therapy itself has been considered traumatic for many Asian Americans: "To share one's problems with *one* person was shameful enough; to share with a group was overwhelming" (Toupin, 1980, p. 85).

To date, no conclusive research exists to suggest that one therapeutic model is more preferable than another for treating culturally diverse individuals (Gopaul-McNicol and Brice-Baker, 1998). Whatever approach one chooses, it is not easy to be completely proficient in working with diverse groups. Assistance should be sought in the assessment or treatment of any client whose cultural background or way of life is unfamiliar or considerably different from that of the therapist (Kurasaki et al., 2000).

Indigenous Forms of Intervention Within the United States

Traumatic incidents and their consequences are viewed by traditional societies as inevitable and unavoidable. As a result, grief, stress, and illness must constantly be managed and accommodated at both the individual and group levels. Culture, to some extent, is

adapted to help the community and its
lane and Van der Kolk, 1996).

Cultural customs and practices help i
emotions, regulate their behavior, conne
the social group, and function as syn
1996). According to Higginbotham (198
enous healing that Western methodolog
language, customs, and values of the loc
points to the major deficit of modern ps
ity" (p. 42).

Every ethnic group has transferred t
not all of its main ideologies and practi
Chioino, 2000). Many immigrants and i
underutilize mainstream mental health s
nous healing methods (herbs, spiritualis
first choice for mental health treatmen
Mexican Americans, for example, hav
tional folk medicine in lieu of modern n
cultural isolation, poverty, discriminat
experience, and strong traditions made
selves and their own resources to maint
of their sick" (Trotter and Chavira, 199

Indigenous healing practices are dev
to accommodate the needs of its memb
context, instead of being transported fro
Seiden, and Lam, 2001). Techniques an
ditional healers in developing nations
use in the West. The public has access t
as those offered in herbalist shops whic
ies (Leff, 1981).

Herbs are a significant resource for i
physical nature. The remedial nature an
these herbs is a mystery to Western sci
tributed to the secrecy involving some o
interest shown by pharmacologists (Lef

Herbs are used by many *curanderos*
properties, such as hallucinogens (pey
and stimulants *(yerba del trueno)* to hel
ter and Chavira, 1997). Descriptions an

recorded in books from Mexico and are now being widely distributed among *curanderos.*

Exorcism (a technique used to expel spirits that cause disease, which continues to be practiced by members of the clergy, although infrequently) and possession are still used for the treatment of psychological and physical conditions outside the realms of scientific medicine (Leff, 1981). It is also common practice for traditional healers to enter into states of possession as a means of determining the cause of sickness or treating those who are afflicted. The healer's ability to diagnose is, presumably, enhanced by the spirit that has entered him or her (Leff, 1981). Some indication suggests that a few of these practices have intensified due to the difficulties that ethnic minorities have encountered while trying to adapt in a society that has a tendency to be economically and psychologically stressful or even hostile to new arrivals (Koss-Chioino, 2000).

Although anthropologists have had a long-standing interest in traditional and folk healing, practitioners of psychology and other behavioral sciences did not consider the significance of these practices to ethnic minorities until recently (Koss-Chioino, 2000). These practitioners now find themselves returning to more traditional methods of healing, due to the multitude of non-European survivors of trauma and "their unwillingness for, or lack of understanding of, psychotherapeutic interventions" (Perren-Klinger, 2000, p. 61).

In Asian cultures, treatment methods provided by traditional healers and herbal doctors are often used repeatedly to remedy physical disorders believed to be the patient's prime problem. Mental health professionals are not regarded as effective and are consulted only as a last resort (Lin et al., 1982).

Cambodian religious beliefs play a part in many of Cambodian patients' understanding of their suffering. Monks and traditional healers perform certain healing ceremonies and practices for physical, emotional, and spiritual pain. These include washing clients with holy water, coining (scraping a coin on the skin), and cupping (burning oxygen under a cup and putting it on the skin at the pain site) (Gerber, Nguyen, and Bounkeua, 1999).

"When stress becomes unendurable, the social network of the Hispanic community often provides access to the system of folk healing as a suitable solution" (Ruiz and Langrod, 1976, p. 95). Three popular folk healing systems that are found in the United States are associ-

ated with the three predominant ethnic
bans, and Mexican Americans: *espirit*
curanderismo (Koss-Chioino, 2000).

Espiritismo

- In espiritismo among Hispanics in
  helped to present the problem by an
  the mediums have raised. The medic
  or "spiritual" causes are at fault in
  Langrod, 1976, p. 96).
- The mediums are given spirit mess;
  either "good or molesting spirits" fc
  client a diagnosis, advice, and a pro;
  are prescribed (Koss, 1987).
- The client is also treated with house
  candle lighting, bathing with speci
  amulets to ward off evil (Comas-Dí
  Spiritist healings are open to the
(Ghali, 1977).

Santeria

- One of the most prevalent religious
  physical and mental distress is S;
  comes from West Africa—specifica
  Ibáñez and Parra, 1999). Practitione
  though goodness exists, it is easily
  Chioino, 2000).
- A significant treatment method in
  forces that range from typical every
  tionship problems, to traumas such ;
  assault, or murder. Santeria, thus, b
  of traumatic incidents (Vélez-Ibáñe;

Curanderismo

- A *curandero* has knowledge of the
  ual, and social worlds. For traumat
  ment method is similar to behavioral
  an automobile accident, the curande

visit the scene of the accident, and after reciting certain prayers and dispelling formulas, the curandero would choose some artifacts from the site including soil if any was around (Vélez-Ibáñez and Parra, 1999).

- Therapeutic sessions would follow, as well as *barrida* (a sweeping), which involves making brushing movements or sweeping the client from head to toe with a lemon, egg, herb, or other appropriate item (Trotter and Chavira, 1997). Barrida is intended to alleviate any psychological stress and literally to "sweep ills away" (Vélez-Ibáñez and Parra, 1999).

While many individuals of African descent are skeptical about their ability to obtain the help they need from Western practitioners, the Western medical system is accepted. Folk remedies passed down through generations are also used (Tully, 1999). Medicines made from plants, herbs, roots, seeds, powders, juices, bones, leaves, minerals, charcoal, and liquids are all used by medicine people in Africa who assume the role of both pastor and doctor in treating afflicted individuals (Mbiti, 1990). Similar medicines have found their place among African-American communities here in the West, as well.

Herbal preparations, sorcery, attendance at spiritual churches, and the rituals of prayer and spiritual cleansing are also elements of traditional practices found in Africa and practiced in Western society (Swartz, 1998; Peddle et al., 1999). The cleansing of one's lifestyle coincides with the process of physical cleansing. Cleansing can be achieved by intense periods of prayer, perhaps, with fasting and sexual abstinence. It may also come in the form of atonement in personal relationships and in a community. People may return to church for cleansing with the guidance of a spiritual leader, friend, or family member (Tully, 1999).

Historically, Caribbean Americans have not been primary consumers of psychological services. Indigenous practices (e.g., obeah, voodoo, espiritismo, and Santeria) provide an adjunctive source of spiritual guidance to Western belief systems such as Catholicism and Protestantism (Gopaul-McNicol and Brice-Baker, 1998). Practitioners of these non-Western belief systems are consulted by Caribbeans for many of the same reasons people seek psychotherapy. They may provide medicinal treatments (herbal preparations); insight into the spiritual forces that may be forming the basis of the person's anxi-

ety; or working spells on the individua
the stress (Gopaul-McNicol and Brice

> Whether demons are within or
> mind is powerful and research d
> influences both the mind and the
> to analyze the safety of traditiona
> people hold traditional cultural b
> tional distress and value their cu
> recognize the longstanding eff
> within the community. (Dubrow

It is also important to appreciate in
mal behavior and curative procedures t
health services effectively to ethnic m
Kohn, and Lee, 2000). Combining tra
current psychological interventions ca
(Dubrow and Nader, 1999).

For many ethnic clients, however,
role ambiguities, language difficulties,
ities, etc., work together to create a rap
cess in therapy (Sue and Zane, 1987).

A study by Flaskerud and Liu (1991
utilization of therapy among ethnic c
would need to be staffed by therapists
language as the clients in the commun
gual and bicultural therapists is especia
cent immigrants and are not fully prof
Wohl, 2000) or for any client who do
mary language (Sue et al., 1991).

Tharp (1991) states that treatment pr
rier is central in the delivery of services
It is not always possible to secure a bi
pecially for languages which are not co
McNicol and Brice-Baker, 1998). Und
health agencies may need to employ t
preters.

Recommended guidelines for the use of a translator-interpreter follow:

- Whenever possible, translators should be professionals rather than family and friends, or office staff (Gopaul-McNicol and Brice-Baker, 1998).
- Translations should be verbatim, and edited summations of the client's words should be avoided (Gopaul-McNicol and Brice-Baker, 1998).
- The interpreter should be familiar with the client's culture (Marcos, 1979).
- The interpreter should be competent in both languages (Marcos, 1979).
- The interpreter should be sensitive and able to work as a team member (Westermeyer, 1990).
- The interpreter should be familiar with psychiatric assessment and care (Westermeyer, 1990).

SUMMARY

1. The goals of psychodynamic therapy are to help the child remember the traumatic event safely; to express any frightening thoughts and feelings associated with those events; and to develop coping skills.
2. Play therapy allows the child to communicate his or her fears without placing too much emphasis on verbalization.
3. Cognitive-behavioral therapy consists of teaching individuals how to cope with anxiety (e.g., deep-breathing exercises, stress-reducing activities) and negative thoughts, as well as anger management.
4. The major behavioral methods utilized in the treatment of individuals diagnosed with PTSD include the following: exposure therapies, systematic desensitization, and stress inoculation.
5. The type of format that a clinician uses in CBT is largely determined by the nature of the traumatic event (e.g., rape, automobile accident, and homicide).
6. Group therapy is often used when large numbers of children are exposed to a common traumatic incident.

7. Debriefings offer survivors oppor
   matic experiences and develop mc
   happened.
8. The entire family is affected when
   posed to a traumatic incident and s
   family therapy may involve all men
9. Medication can help older childr
   anxiety, depression, and insomnia
10. Interventions may work best in sc
    comfortable, and natural environm
11. There has been agreement, for the
    stress appears to be universal (Marse
12. As cultural and ethnic diversities in
    does the need for specific modes o
13. It is important that family therapy
    attributes of the extended family s
14. Every ethnic group has transferred
    not all, of its main ideologies and
    (Koss-Chioino, 2000).
15. Techniques and remedies employe
    tinue to have widespread use in the
16. Herbs are a significant resource for
    physical nature.

Chapter 5

Establishing a School-Based Trauma Response Team

Most educators do not enter the profession expecting to help students and staff respond in the face of a tragedy. However, in reality, when a school-based crisis presents, meeting the needs of the school family calls for the collaborative effort of *all* educators. (Lerner, Volpe, and Lindell, 2003, p. 89)

Too often, children are the victims of traumatic incidents. If trauma were to strike, its impact would most likely be felt in schools where many children happen to congregate.

BOX 5.1.
Examples of Traumatic Incidents in a School Setting

- A student is accosted by a male intruder in the rest room and is sexually assaulted.
- The administrative assistant receives a bomb threat over the telephone, and the entire school has to be evacuated immediately.
- Four students, under the influence of alcohol, are killed in an automobile accident following the school prom.
- A school shooting, started by some students who were expelled the previous day, claims the lives of four students and a teacher.
- A school bus transporting fifteen students and two faculty members on a field trip is taken hostage by a deranged gunman.
- A hurricane causes severe damage to school property and surrounding neighborhoods.
- A teacher's aide is accused of sexually molesting two preschoolers.

Educators and other professional car
called upon to help students, school
with the emotional stress reactions ass
loss, or accidental death. It is not enou
skills of a school administrator or guid
cidents require the emergency planning
eral trained and available members of t
ing outside resources.

The need for careful planning before
rence of a traumatic incident is absolu
dress this need is to establish a traun
1992; Moriarty, Maeyama, and Fitzge
Trauma response teams are a partnershi
fessionals and other helping profession
itating the prevention of posttraumatic
cidents, homicides, suicides, terrorism,
that occur in much of the world.

Currently more than 300 formal tr
place across the globe. The critical inc
was utilized and applied to high-risk c
law enforcement, emergency medicine,
personnel, and disaster response (Mitc
subsequently been adopted by other occ
clergy, military, corporations, and scho

A school-based trauma response tea
following:

- School administrators (principal,
- School social worker/counselor/ps
- School nurse
- Head teacher
- Security officer
- School secretary

Other participants, such as representative
portation departments, may be selecte
needs of the school.

The TRT has many functions, some o
a traumatic incident, the team should pe

- *Decide who will be in charge* during a traumatic incident. The person chosen may be the school principal. If so, he will have to be available at all times and, therefore, may have to assign his usual administrative duties to an assistant. It is also important to choose a backup person, if the principal or other appointed leader is unavailable at the time of the traumatic incident.
- *Develop a trauma response plan* before a traumatic incident strikes. This allows the TRT to make as many decisions as possible while things are calm.
- *Prepare and review board policies and procedures* related to traumatic incidents for their consistency and completeness. It is important that specific guidelines outline the functions and responsibilities of faculty during an emergency.
- *Assess the trauma response plan* for consistency and ease of implementation.
- *Prepare faculty* for what to expect during a traumatic incident.
- *Train faculty* in understanding their assigned roles and how to intervene during a traumatic incident.
- *Involve other helping professionals* in the trauma response plan—such as the local police and fire department—so they may know of your preparations and offer their expertise. Phone numbers of the local police, fire, health, and social service departments should be readily accessible in the school office.
- *Periodically review* the team's response to a traumatic incident for quality assurance.

All members of the TRT must be trained in trauma response and have full knowledge of their roles and responsibilities in following procedures outlined in the plan. Members need to have an understanding of the various types of trauma that may strike the school and how to respond to children's reactions, as well as those of faculty. Ongoing training should be provided on topics such as traumatic stress, grief and loss, child abuse, suicide, conflict resolution, coping strategies, first aid, and referral. The trauma response team should consider the following questions:

> What are the training needs of the members?
> When, how, and where will the training be provided?
> Should training include all faculty members?

RESPONSIBL.
OF THE TRAUMA RE.

The school principal has the key ro
assigning various functions to team me
by community members as the one in
her to restore order in times of crisis. T
however. It is the TRT as a whole th
sponse plan into action.

Responsibilities of the School Princi

- Maintain a high profile (Thomas.
- Maintain ongoing communicatio
  dent's office (Thomas, 1993).
- Mobilize the TRT.
- Maintain a list of the day and
  members to carry at all times (Ja
- Obtain legal counsel (Jay, 1989).
- Identify students and faculty who
- Inform faculty on how to address
  incident.
- Assign school representatives to
  jured or deceased.
- Consider methods of addressing
  tions.
- Decide what information is to be
- Arrange for visits to the familie
  ceased.
- Arrange for faculty to attend gro
- Inform faculty and parents of
  school.
- Be responsible for rumor control
- Provide crowd management.

Responsibilities of the Vice Principal

- Assist the principal with adminis
  lated to the traumatic incident.
- Offer assistance to the principal in
  sibilities.

- Substitute for the principal if he or she is not available during a traumatic incident.

Responsibilities of the Counseling Professional (Guidance Counselor, School Social Worker, or School Psychologist)

- Coordinate counseling activities. This includes serving as an intermediary between the school and mental health systems, assessing high-risk students immediately following a traumatic incident, evaluation, family contact, referral, and follow-up as necessary.
- Understand developmentally based reactions to trauma.
- Recruit outside help for more detailed assessment and treatment of high-risk students, if needed.
- Help with the logistics of the debriefing and counseling activities.
- Obtain a list from teachers of those students requesting counseling services.
- Coordinate the return of survivors to school after hospitalization.

Responsibilities of the School Nurse

- Help to administer first aid and cardiopulmonary resuscitation (CPR) as necessary.
- Assist with the logistics of the aid and transport of victims needing medical care.

Responsibility of the Head Teacher

- Serve as a team liaison to faculty.

Responsibility of the Security Officer

- Help provide safety instructions, and plan to ensure protection of everyone involved.

BOX 5.2. Equipment

TRT Members

Backpack, gloves, helmet, heavy clc
light with extra batteries, whistle, w
pens, copy of disaster plan, emergenc
duct tape, utility shutoff tools, first-aic

Teachers

First-aid supplies and instructions, ba
ies, whistle, paper, pens, scissors,
large plastic garbage bags, hard canc
per cups, toilet paper, medical relea
dents' parent release forms (includir
are authorized to pick specific stude
cards, a copy of the disaster plan, a b
debris and broken glass

Administrative Assistant(s)

Spiral notebook to keep records of th
per pad, pens, copy of the disaster pl
radio, extra batteries, walkie-talkie

Principal

Paper pad, pens, a copy of the disaste
talkie, extra batteries, bull horn, whis1

Designated Staff Person

Students' medications

Nurse

Adhesive strips (plastic), triangular k
dages, sterile gauze pads, instant cc
petroleum jelly, antibiotic ointment, s

(continued)

able gloves (latex), antiseptic wipes, soap, medicine cups, toilet paper, ice bags, safety pins of assorted sizes, alcohol, cotton tip applicators, cotton balls, tongue depressors, tweezers, scissors, first-aid cream, hydrogen peroxide, ipecac, paper towels, saline, sterile eye pads, eyewash, stretch gauze bandage (Ace type), cervical collar (various sizes), disposable thermometers, bulb syringe, blood pressure cuff with manometer, disposable splints, needle and thread, plastic trash bags, tissues, penlight with battery, sanitary napkins, blankets, stretcher

School Bus/Maintenance Vehicles

AM/FM radio, jumper cables, rope for towing or rescue, fire extinguisher, first-aid kit, tool kit, road map, compass, shovel, sack of sand, leather work gloves, flashlight or signal light with extra batteries, plastic scraper, duct tape, plastic sheeting, list of emergency phone numbers, tire chains (in areas with heavy snow)

Other Recommended Equipment and Supplies

Shovels (square, round point, and collapsible), wrecking bar, nylon rope, air horn or bell, answering machine, radio (solar or battery), lights/lanterns, megaphone, hard hat, safety goggles, wrenches to turn off gas valves, cellular phone

TRAUMA RESPONSE TEAM CHECKLIST

Assembling the TRT

The TRT should convene as soon as possible following a traumatic incident. Compile a list of each team member's name and available phone numbers, and gather any factual information concerning the incident from the local police, fire, and rescue departments.

Announcing the Incident to Faculty (Armistead, 1996)

- Decide how, where, and when the incident will be announced.
- Decide what method will be used to contact faculty (e.g., phone tree).
- Decide who will make the announcement.

Announcing the Incident to Students

- Decide how, where, and when the
- Decide what method will be used
- Decide who will make the annou

Managing the Media

- Assign a media spokesperson. (*A* backup.)

Responding to Outside Calls

- Assign people to log all phone ca decide what should or should not

Reporting the Incident to the Police

- Assign a person to handle com and/or fire and rescue department

Communicating to Family Members

- Assign a person to address the co

Functions of the Faculty

Teachers

- Facilitate classroom discussion o gestions in Chapter 4).
- Identify students at risk.
- Inform school counselors' office c services.

- Create activities for classroom involvement to help students cope with the incident (see list of possible activities in Chapter 4).
- Cancel any scheduled assignments for a few days. If this is not possible, try to shorten the length and structure the assignments.
- Postpone any scheduled exams.
- Inform students of any plans regarding a memorial service and/or funeral for the victims. Prepare students for attendance.

Administrative Assistant(s)

- Arrange for additional secretarial support, if needed.
- Prevent any student activity reports from being sent to the home of parents whose child has died.
- Maintain ongoing communications with faculty.
- Establish transportation and arrange for any excused absences for students who wish to attend a funeral.
- Provide factual information concerning the incident.

Counseling Department

- Be available to offer assistance to any student or faculty member at risk.
- Provide supportive counseling to any student or faculty member needing or requesting services.
- Recruit additional resources, if needed.
- Keep a record of those students who received counseling, for follow-up purposes.
- Conduct counseling groups for those students affected by the incident.

Meeting with the Victims' Families

Assign school representatives to visit the families of those seriously injured or deceased. (The school principal should make the initial visit with the families and then assign school representatives to those families in need of additional follow-up.) The victims' families are to be contacted as soon as possible and practical. Plan to address any language or cultural differences beforehand.

Purposes of the Family Visit

- Communicate the needs and conce
- Offer comfort to the families.
- Demonstrate the concerns and car
- Find out the wishes of the family.
- Learn the logistics of the facility h
  plan for student transportation anc
  family wishes for students to be p

Initiating Contact at the Homes of Fa

- Phone the parents of the victim to
  visit.
- Be aware of any signs of anger dir
  ing for the visit may not be appro

Initiating Contact with Families at the

Call the hospital and arrange ahead o
in a private room, if available. The wai
cially if several family members are pr

PREPARING FOR T

Educators often find themselves the f
a traumatic incident strikes their schoo
proper preparation, however, this too sl

- Select a specific spokesperson anc
  to respond to the media during a
  (Thomas, 1993).
- Obtain training on how to deal effect
  1993).
- Establish good relations with repor
  any traumatic incident (Potter, 199
- Be knowledgeable of board polic
  tions, and the school district's pc
  tions.

- Maintain accurate and up-to-date mailing labels for families of students.
- Make sure student information files are updated, including emergency contact information.
- Designate an area in your school to serve as a "communications command center" and direct all media there (Crawford, 1992).
- Brainstorm with the TRT about all the possible questions reporters might ask and responses you will provide (Potter, 1997).

BOX 5.3. Media Relations Checklist

Dealing with the Media

- Make sure you have all the facts before responding to the media (Wayne, 1992).
- Return phone calls promptly (Williams, 1993).
- Be available at all times to reporters who arrive on the scene or who telephone.
- Give the media a phone number to reach you after hours.
- Tell the truth (Williams, 1993).
- Avoid saying "no comment." Refer a reporter to someone else with more information, such as the police (Wayne, 1992).
- Be positive, not defensive (Wayne, 1992).
- Deal with the facts. Don't give your personal opinions.
- Don't blame others for school problems (Potter, 1997).
- Take a deep breath and count to ten if you get angry (Wayne, 1992).
- Do not be elusive.
- Keep your language simple; avoid jargon.
- Do not use humor under serious circumstances (Potter, 1997).
- It is all right to say you don't know.
- Choose your words and phrases with caution.
- Be aware of your body language.
- Do not provide information and then comment that it is "off the record" (Williams, 1993).
- If you are unsure of an answer, take a phone number and call back rather than risk giving the wrong answer.
- Notify school staff and board of all facts—to keep them informed—and dispel any false rumors.

(continued)

(continued)

Rumor Control

- Arrange before- and/or after-schoo
  rate information to staff.
- Be available to address any conce
  rive to pick up their children.
- Send home fliers to parents to p
  school is managing the traumatic i
- Provide a script for administrativ
  sponding to questions from curiou:
- Log all incoming calls.
- Always keep the school superinten
  members updated.
- Obtain all facts of the incident rega
  when, and the consequences for re
- Establish a telephone tree and di
  signed to making phone calls.
- Update students periodically in the
- Designate a media spokesperson ;
  son.
- Establish a police liaison who can
  exchange relevant information (M
  gerald, 1993).
- Establish a code number or name
  public address system to alert staf
  matic incident without creating cha

FACULTY AND STAFF GR(

Debriefings have been shown to h
term effects that are associated with tr
to help individuals gain insight and beg
cident from a different and more helpf

In a debriefing, the faculty and staff
were affected by the traumatic incident
vate location. Ground rules are establi
couraged to share their experiences.

Group debriefings should normally occur within seventy-two hours of the traumatic incident and are usually led by a mental health professional.

Your debriefings should provide the following:

- Resolution of any misperceptions
- Education
- Cohesion
- Sharing and validation of emotions
- Encouragement and support
- Improved communications
- Screening for those in need of counseling

Setting up the Debriefing

Who

- School faculty and staff directly involved in the incident
- School faculty and staff who actually witnessed the incident
- School faculty and staff who may have been marginally exposed to the incident
- School faculty and staff who were absent by chance
- A separate debriefing can be arranged for the principal, vice principal, and the rest of the TRT
- No media or outsiders allowed

It is recommended that debriefings be mandatory for affected faculty and staff as a preventive measure and to ensure that they get the help they need.

Develop a procedure for informing faculty and staff of the time and place of the debriefing. Find out the number of faculty and staff to be debriefed. Consider dividing up the group if more than fifteen participants are present. Make sure enough mental health professionals are on hand to cover the debriefings. Also make sure that the school counselor/social worker/psychologist has enough time to attend to those faculty and staff needing individual supportive counseling. Plan for additional resources if necessary.

Where

- A safe and neutral place away fro
  tion
- A room that can accommodate u
- Sufficient climate and lighting
- No devices that make noise (e.g.,
- Restricted access
- No outside interruptions or distu

When

- Arrange times for debriefings. Re
  meeting.

It will most likely be a long and em
ticipants. Consider having light, nutrit

SUMMAR

1. One way educators can handle a t
   trauma response team (TRT).
2. Currently more than 300 formal
   place across the globe.
3. All members of the TRT must be t
   have full knowledge of their roles
   ing procedures outlined in the plar
4. Ongoing training should be provid
   stress, grief and loss, child abuse
   coping strategies, first aid, and ref
5. The TRT may consist of school
   workers, counselors, psychologists
   security officers, school secretarie
6. The school principal has the key ro
   assigning various functions to tear
7. The TRT should convene as soon
   matic incident.
8. Debriefings have been shown to h
   term effects that are associated wit

9. In a debriefing, the faculty and staff members of your school who were affected by the traumatic incident are invited to convene in a private location. Ground rules are established, and participants are encouraged to share their experiences.
10. Group debriefings should normally occur within seventy-two hours of the traumatic incident and are usually led by a mental health professional.
11. It is recommended that debriefings be mandatory for affected faculty and staff as a preventive measure and to ensure that they get the help they need.
12. It is important that your students be given the opportunity to express their feelings and ask questions which may be helpful in alleviating any fears or concerns they may have.
13. Teach your students appropriate ways they can cope and manage their stress. Inform them of any counseling activities that are to take place in the school.

Epilogu

Up from a past that's rootec
Leaving behind night of ter

A country that neglects its own chi
pride, only shame. A country that refu.
to lend aid to those who are suffering n
stretched out. Children, whether your o
to be cared for in a nurturing environme
cal and psychological harm, and afforc
all human beings, including the right t(

Children from every corner of the v
great deal in their young lives. They ma}
ors and even behave beyond their years
enced a true sense of childhood. Nevertl

That unsuspecting person being hurl
That frightened person posing nude be
innocent person being belittled and tort
person sleeping on the sidewalk *is a cl*
ning across a minefield *is a child.* That c
is a child. That faceless person in the gr;
every one of us is a child who just wan

We are not living in a different worl
only more exposed. Our dirty laundry i
closed doors. It is scattered out onto th«
either close our eyes, look the other wa}
can collectively gather it up and begin

Trauma will always be present in the
tinue to give birth. As caregivers, we w
tant role in shaping the lives of those chi

We will show them that, in the face of trauma, growth and healing can occur; knowledge and awareness can be found; love and forgiveness can be achieved; peace and hope can be restored; and another way and a new beginning can be devised. There can be a future.

Resourc

BOOKS, CURRICULA, AND ▮

Readings for Administrators, Teacher and Health Care Practitioners

Apfel, Roberta and Simon, Bennett (Eds.) (199
  Mental Health of Children in War and Con
  Yale University Press.
Beane, Allan L. and Espeland, Pamela (1999). *7*
  Tips and Strategies for Teachers K-8. Minne
Begun, Ruth W. and Huml, Frank F. (Eds.) (200
  tion Skills, Lessons, and Activities for El
  Jossey-Bass.
Carlson-Paige, Nancy and Levin, Diane E. (19
  Building Conflict Resolution Skills with Chil
Curcio, Joan L. and First, Patricia F. (1993).
  Proactively Prevent and Defuse it (Roadma
  ministrator's Leadership). Thousand Oaks, ▮
Dennison, Susan T. and Knight, Connie M. (19
  apy: A Guide for Planning and Facilitating
  Springfield, IL: Charles C. Thomas Pub. Ltc
Eth, Spencer and Pynoos, Robert S. (Eds.) (198
  in Children. Arlington, VA: American Psycl
Ewing, Charles (1995). *Kids Who Kill.* New Yc
Fead, A. K. (1985). *Child Abuse Crisis: Impact c*
Gil, Eliana (1991). *The Healing Power of Pla*
  New York: Guilford Press.
Girard, Kathy and Koch, Susan J. (1996). *Cor*
  Manual for Educators (Jossey-Bass Educa*
  Dispute Resolution. Somerset, NJ: Jossey-B*
Goldstein, Arnold P. and Kodluboy, Donald W
  Symbols, and Solutions. Champaign, IL: Res
Goodwin-Gill, Guy S. and Cohen, Ilene (19
  Children in Armed Conflict. New York: Oxf
Green, Arthur H. (1980). *Child Maltreatment: ▮*
  Child Care Professionals. Northvale, NJ: Ja*

Hicks, Barbara Barret (1990). *Youth Suicide: A Comprehensive Manual for Prevention and Intervention.* Bloomington, IN: National Educational Service.

Hill, Marie Somers and Hill, Frank W. (1994). *Creating Safe Schools: What Principals Can Do (Principals Taking Action).* Thousand Oaks, CA: Corwin Press.

Kivel, Paul, Creighton, Allan, and Oakland Men's Project (1996). *Making the Peace: A 15-Session Violence Prevention Curriculum for Young People.* Alameda, CA: Hunter House.

Lafromboise, Teresa Davis (1996). *American Indian Life Skills Development Curriculum.* Madison: University of Wisconsin Press.

Lantieri, Linda and Patti, Janet (1998). *Waging Peace in Our Schools.* Boston, MA: Beacon Press.

Miller, Maryann (1999). *Weapons and Violence at Schools and on Your Streets (Coping).* New York: Rosen Publishing Group.

Ramsey, Robert D. (1994). *Administrator's Complete School Discipline Guide: Techniques and Materials for Creating an Environment Where Kids Can Learn.* Upper Saddle River, NJ: Prentice-Hall.

Rose, Steven R. (1998). *Group Work with Children and Adolescents: Prevention and Intervention in School and Community Systems* (Sage Sourcebooks for the Human Services, vol. 38). Thousand Oaks, CA: Sage Publications.

Rubel, Barbara (2000). *But I Didn't Say Goodbye: For Parents and Professionals Helping Child Suicide Survivors.* Kendall Park, NJ: Griefwork Center.

Schmidt, Teresa and Lindberg Design (1993). *Anger Management: A Group Activities Manual for Middle and High School Students.* Minneapolis, MN: Johnson Institute—QVS.

Taylor, Barbara J. (1998). *A Child Goes Forth: A Curriculum Guide for Preschool Children* (Ninth Edition). Upper Saddle River, NJ: Prentice-Hall.

Terr, Lenore (1990). *Too Scared to Cry: Psychic Trauma in Childhood* (First Edition). New York: Harper and Row.

Trad, Paul V. (1990). *Treating Suicidelike Behavior in a Preschooler.* Guilford, CT: International Universities Press.

Video Programs

The Bureau for At-Risk Youth, In-service training videos on topics such as death and grief, suicide prevention, school violence, and more. *Elementary, Middle School, and Teen Guidance Videos; Violence Prevention Videos.* 1-800-99-YOUTH.

J. Gary Mitchell Film Company, Video Programs on Child Abuse Prevention. *What Tadoo; What Tadoo with Secrets; Believe Me.* 1-800-301-4050.

J. Gary Mitchell Film Company, Video Programs on Violence Prevention. *No Means No; Words Can Hurt; A Friend in Need.* 1-800-301-4050.

Children's Books on Natural Disaste
(Ages Four to Eight)

Beatty, Monica D. (1999). *Fire Night!* Oxforc

Bridwell, Norman (1995). *Clifford and the Bi*
  Madison, WI: Demco Media.

Cole, Joanna (1996). *The Magic School Bus Ir*
  Series). New York: Scholastic Trade.

Enderle, Judith A. (1996). *Francis, the Ea*
  Chronicle Books.

Lewis, Thomas P. (1997). *La Montana De F*
  York: Harper Trophy.

Milne, A. A. (1997). *Pooh to the Rescue/Bc*
  Blocks. New York: Penguin USA.

Parker, M. J. (1990). *City Storm.* New York: $

Sloat, Teri (2001). *Farmer Brown Goes Rou*
  Merchandise.

Van Allsburg, Chris (1997). *Ben's Dream.* B
  pany.

Velthuijs, Max (1996). *Frog Is a Hero.* Londc

Children's Books on Natural Disaste
(Ages Nine to Twelve)

Billings, Henry (1990). *Great Disasters.* Orlai

Carter, Alden R. (1994). *Dogwolf.* New York:

Cooney, Caroline B. (1995). *Flash Fire.* New

Cottonwood, Joe (1995). *Quake! A Novel.* Ne

Garland, Sherry (1995). *The Silent Storm.* San

Haas, Jessie (1998). *Fire! My Parents' Story.*

Lowell, Susan (1993). *I Am Lavina Cumming*
  tions.

Mark, Bonnie S. (1997). *I'll Know What to Do.*
  Washington, DC: Magination.

Mitchell, Nancy (1999). *Earth Rising. Book*
  Fremont, CA: Lightstream Publications.

Mitchell, Nancy (1999). *Raging Skies. Book*
  Fremont, CA: Lightstream Publications.

Nicolson, Cynthia P. (2002). *Earthquake.* Tor

Children's Books on Violence—Child Abuse, Suicide, Bullying, War, and Terrorism (Ages Four to Eight)

Chaiet, Donna and Russell, Francine (1998). *The Safe Zone: A Kid's Guide to Personal Safety.* New York: William Morrow and Company.

Goldman, Linda E. (1998). *Bart Speaks Out: Breaking the Silence on Suicide.* Los Angeles, CA: Western Psychological Services.

Hopkins, Beverly H. (2001). *My Mom Has a Bad Temper.* Washington, DC: Child Welfare League of America.

Jackson, Ellen and Rotner, Shelley (2002). *Sometimes Bad Things Happen* (Single Titles). Riverside, NJ: Millbrook Press Trade.

Julik, Edie (2000). *Sailing Through the Storm: To the Ocean of Peace.* Lakeville, MN: Galde Press.

Kleven, Sandy (1998). *The Right Touch: A Read-Aloud Story to Help Prevent Child Sexual Abuse.* Bellevue, WA: Illumination Arts.

Lobel, Anita (2000). *No Pretty Pictures: A Child of War.* Tampa, FL: Camelot.

Spelman, Cornelia (1997). *Your Body Belongs to You.* Morton Grove, IL: Albert Whitman and Company.

Children's Books on Violence—Child Abuse, Suicide, Bullying, War, and Terrorism (Ages Nine to Twelve)

Banks, Lynne Reid (1999). *Maura's Angel.* Tampa, FL: Camelot.

Ewing, Lynne (1998). *Drive By.* New York: Harpercollins Juvenile Books.

Gow, Mary (2002). *Attack on America: The Day the Twin Towers Collapsed.* Berkeley Heights, NJ: Enslow.

Martin, Ann M. (1998). *Claudia and the Terrible Truth* (Baby-Sitters Club, No. 117). Hermitage, TN: Apple.

Tabor, Nancy (1999). *Bottles Break.* Watertown, MA: Charlesbridge Publishing.

Temple, Frances (1994). *Taste of Salt: A Story of Modern Haiti.* New York: Harper Trophy.

Wynn-Jones, Tim (1998). *The Maestro.* London: Puffin.

Children's Books on Violence—Child Abuse, Suicide, Bullying, War, and Terrorism (Ages Thirteen to Eighteen)

Nye, Naomi Shihab (Ed.) (1998). *The Space Between Our Footsteps: Poems and Paintings From the Middle East.* Riverside, NJ: Simon and Schuster.

Palmer, Jed (1994). *Everything You Need To K*
  lent Crime (The Need To Know Library S
  Group.
Tolan, Stephanie S. (2000). *Welcome to the A*
Trottier, Maxine (1997). *A Safe Place.* Mor
  Company.
Velasquez, Gloria (1998). *Rina's Family Sec*
  Houston, TX: Arte Publico Press.
Yee, John W. (1997). *The Bully Buster Book (*
  ume 1). Toronto, Ontario: Outgoing Press.

Children's Books on Grief (Ages For

De Paola, Tomie (2000). *Nana Upstairs and I*
Gish, Louise and Rothman, Juliet C. (1996)
  Child's Story of Loss. Amherst, NY: Prom
Jukes, Mavis (2002). *I'll See You in My Drea*
Kidd, Diana (1991). *Onion Tears.* Guilford, L
Moser, Adolph (1998). *Don't Despair on*
  Management Book (The Emotional Impact
  Editions.
Szaj, Kathleen C. (1997). *I Hate Goodbyes.* N
Williams, Carol Lynch (1996). *Adeline Stree*
  pany.
Winsch, Jane L. (1995). *After the Funeral.* M

Children's Books on Grief (Ages Nin

Moser, Adolph (1998). *Don't Despair on*
  Management Book (The Emotional Impact
  Editions.
Romain, Trevor and Verdick, Elizabeth (1999
  Someone Dies? Minneapolis, MN: Free Sp
Rothman, Juliet C. (1996). *A Birthday Presen*
  Amherst, NY: Prometheus Books.
Stevens, Diane (1997). *Liza's Star Wish.* New

Children's Books on Grief (Ages Thi

Grollman, Earl A. (1993). *Straight Talk Abou*
  with Losing Someone You Love. Boson, M

CRISIS HOTLINE NUMBERS

Abuses of Children's Human Rights

Human Rights Hotline
Hotline fax number in Geneva: 41-22-917-0092
Hours: 24-hour facsimile line
Who: victims of human rights violations, their relatives, and nongovernmental organizations

Auto Safety

Department of Transportation Auto Safety Hotline
1-888-DASH-2-DOT
1-888-327-4236

Child Abuse

Childhelp USA (National Child Abuse Hotline)
800-4A Child (800-422-4453)
Hours: 24 hours 7 days
Who: child abuse victims, offenders, parents

Youth Crisis Hotline (Youth Development International)
800-Hit-Home (800-448-4663)
Hours: 24 hours 7 days
Who: individuals reporting child abuse

Family Violence

National Domestic Violence Hotline
800-799-SAFE (800-799-7233)
Hours: 24 hours 7 days
Who: children, parents, friends, offenders

Missing/Abducted Children

Child Find of America
800-I AM LOST (800-426-5678)
Hours: 9-5 EST, M-F; 24-hour answering machine
Who: parents reporting lost or abducted children

Child Find of America Mediation
800-A Way Out (800-292-9688)
Hours: 9-5 EST, M-F; 24-hour answering r
Who: parents (abduction, child custody)

Child Quest International Sighting Line
888-818-4673
Hours: 24 hours 7 days
Who: individuals with a missing child, emer

Operation Lookout National Center for Mis
800-782-SEEK (800-782-7335)
Hours: 24 hours 7 days
Who: individuals with a missing child, emer

Rape/Incest

Rape Abuse and Incest National Network (
800-656-HOPE (800-656-4673)
Hours: 24 hours 7 days
Who: rape and incest victims

Relief for Caregivers

National Respite Locator Service
800-7-RELIEF (800-773-5433)
Hours: 8:30-5:00 EST, M-F
Who: parents and professionals caring for c
illness, or at risk of child abuse or neglect

Victims of Violent Crimes

Arson Hotline
888-ATF-FIRE (888-283-3473)

Bomb Hotline
888-ATF-BOMB (888-283-2662)

National Center for Victims of Crime
800-FYI-CALL (800-394-2255)
Hours: 8:30-5:30 EST, M-F
Who: all victims of violent crimes

Youth in Trouble/Runaways

Covenant House Hotline
800-999-9999
Hours: 24 hours 7 days
Who: problem teens and runaways, family members

Girls and Boys Town
800-448-3000
Hours: 24 hours 7 days
Who: troubled children, parents, family members

National Referral Network for Kids in Crisis
800-KID-SAVE (800-543-7283)
Hours: 24 hours 7 days
Who: professionals, parents, adolescents

National Runaway Switchboard (NRS)
800-621-4000
Hours: 24 hours 7 days
Who: adolescents, families

Youth Crisis Hotline (Youth Development International)
800-Hit-Home (800-448-4663)
Hours: 24 hours 7 days
Who: individuals wishing to obtain help for runaways

ORGANIZATIONS

American Academy of Experts in Traumatic Stress
  Administrative offices:
  368 Veterans Memorial Highway
  Commack, NY 11725
  631-543-2217

American Psychiatric Association
  1400 K. Street, N.W.
  Washington, DC 20005
  Answer Center: 202-682-6000

American Psychological Association
   750 First Street, N.E.
   Washington, DC 20002-4242
   800-374-2721

American Red Cross National Headquarters
   2025 E. Street, N.W.
   Washington, DC 20006
   202-303-4498

Amnesty International, USA
   322 Eighth Avenue
   New York, NY 10001
   212-807-8400

Association of Traumatic Stress Specialists
   P.O. Box 2747
   Georgetown, TX 78627
   512-868-3677

Center for the Prevention of School Violence
   1801 Mail Service Center
   Raleigh, NC 27699-1801
   1-800-299-6054

Centers for Disease Control and Prevention
   1600 Clifton Road
   Atlanta, GA 30333
   800-311-3435

Federal Emergency Management Agency
   Federal Center Plaza
   500 C. Street, S.W.
   Washington, DC 20472
   202-566-1600

Institute for Urban and Minority Education
   Box 75
   Teacher's College, Columbia University
   New York, NY 10027-6696
   212-678-3780

International Committee of the Red Cross
  19 Avenue de la Paix
  CH 1202 Geneve
  ++41(22) 7346001

International Society of Traumatic Stress Studies
  60 Revere Drive, Suite 500
  Northbrook, IL 60062
  847-480-9028

National Association of School Psychologists
  4340 East West Highway
  Suite 402
  Bethesda, MD 20814
  301-657-0270

The National Association of Social Workers
  750 First St., N.E.
  Suite 700
  Washington, DC 20002-4241
  202-408-8600

National Center for Conflict Resolution Education
  110 W. Main Street
  Urbana, IL 61801
  800-308-9419

National Center for Educational Statistics
  1990 K. Street, N.W.
  Washington, DC 20006
  202-502-7300

National Center for Injury Prevention and Control
  Mail Stop K65
  4770 Buford Highway N.E.
  Atlanta, GA 30341-3724
  770-488-1506

National Clearinghouse on Child Abuse and Neglect Information
  330 C Street, S.W.
  Washington, DC 20447
  800-394-3366

National Crime Prevention Council
   1000 Connecticut Avenue, N.W.
   Thirteenth Floor
   Washington, DC 20036
   202-466-6272

National Highway Traffic Safety Administrati
   400 7th St. S.W.
   Washington, DC 20590

National Institute for Mental Health (NIMH)
   Office of Communications
   6001 Executive Boulevard, Rm. 8184
   MSC 9663
   Bethesda, MD 20892-9663
   866-615-6464

National Resource Center for Safe Schools (N
   101 S.W. Main
   Suite 500
   Portland, OR 97204
   1-800-268-2275

National School Safety Center
   141 Duesenberg Drive
   Suite 11
   Westlake Village, CA 91362
   805-373-9977

National Transportation Safety Board
   Public Inquiries Branch
   490 L'enfant Plaza, S.W.
   Washington, DC 20594
   800-877-6799

Natural Hazards Center
   482 UCB
   University of Colorado
   Boulder, CO 80309-0482
   303-492-6818

Office of Juvenile Justice and Delinquency Prevention
    810 Seventh Street, N.W.
    Washington, DC 20531
    202-307-5911

Save the Children
    Attn: Donor Services
    54 Wilton Road
    Westport, CT 06880
    800-728-3843

UCLA School Mental Health Project
    Center for Mental Health in Schools
    Department of Psychology
    PO Box 951563
    Los Angeles, CA 90095-1563
    866-846-4843

United Nations Department of Public Information
    United Nations, Room S-1040
    New York, NY 10017
    212-963-4475

U.S. Committee for UNICEF
    333 East 38th Street
    New York, NY 10016
    800-FOR-KIDS (1-800-367-5437)

U.S. Department of Education
    400 Maryland Avenue, S.W.
    Washington, DC 20202-0498
    800-USA-LEARN (800-872-5327)

U.S. Department of Health and Human Services
    200 Independence Avenue, S.W.
    Washington, DC 20201
    877-696-6775

U.S. Department of Justice
    Office for Victims of Crime
    810 Seventh Street, N.W.
    Washington, DC 20531
    800-851-3420

U.S. Fire Administration
  16825 S. Seton Ave.
  Emmitsburg, MD 21727
  301-447-1000 (voice)

U.S. Geological Survey
  1-888-ASK-USGS (1-888-275-8747)

References

Abudabbeh, N. (1994). Treatment of post-traumatic stress disorder in the Arab-American community. In M. B. Williams and J. F. Sommer Jr. (Eds.), *Handbook of post-traumatic therapy* (pp. 252-267). Westport, CT: Greenwood Press.

Ahmad, A., Sofi, M. A., Sundelin-Wahlsten, V., von Knorring, A. L. (2000). Posttraumatic stress disorder in children after the military operation "Anfal" in Iraqi Kurdistan. *European Child and Adolescent Psychiatry, 9,* 235-243.

Ajdukovic, M. (1998). Displaced adolescents in Croatia: Sources of stress and posttraumatic stress reaction. *Adolescence, 33,* 209-217.

American Psychiatric Association (1987). *Diagnostic and statistical manual of mental disorders* (Third edition, Revised). Washington, DC: American Psychiatric Association.

American Psychiatric Association (1994). *Diagnostic and statistical manual of mental disorders* (Fourth edition). Washington, DC: American Psychiatric Association.

Amnesty International United Kingdom (1999). *In the firing line: War and children's rights.* London: Author.

Angelou, M. (1978). *And still I rise* (First edition). New York: Random House.

Aponte, J. F. and Wohl, J. (Eds.) (2000). *Psychological intervention and cultural diversity* (Second edition). Boston: Allyn and Bacon.

Armistead, L. (1996). What to do before the violence happens: Designing the crisis communication plan. *NAASP Bulletin, 80,* 31-37.

Arroyo, W. and Eth, S. (1996). Post-traumatic stress disorder and other stress reactions. In R. J. Apfel and B. Simon (Eds.), *Minefields in their hearts: The mental health of children in war and communal violence* (pp. 52 - 74). New Haven: Yale University Press.

Awwad, E. (1999). Between trauma and recovery: Some perspectives on Palestinian's vulnerability and adaptation. In K. Nader, N. Dubrow, and B. H. Stamm (Eds.), *The series in trauma and loss: Honoring differences: Cultural issues in the treatment of trauma and loss* (pp. 234-265). Philadelphia: Brunner/Mazel.

Azarian, A. G., Lipsitt, L. P., Miller, T. W., and Skriptchenko-Gregorian, V. G. (1999). Toddlers remember quake trauma. In L. M. Williams and V. L. Banyard (Eds.), *Trauma and memory* (pp. 299-310). Thousand Oaks, CA: Sage Publications.

Bauer, P. J. (1997). Development of memory in early childhood. In N. Cowan (Ed.), *The development of memory in childhood* (pp. 83-111). London: Psychology Press.

Bemak, F. P. and Chung, R. C. (2000). Psycho
and refugees. In J. F. Aponte and J. Wohl (E
cultural diversity (Second edition) (pp. 20C

Berk, L. E. (2000). *Child development* (Fifth e

Birchard, K. (1998). Suicides in Ireland increa

Blom, G. E. (1986). A school disaster—Interv
of the American Academy of Child Psychia

Bodley, J. H. (1997). *Cultural anthropology:*
(Second edition). Mountain View, CA: Ma

Bolea, P. S., Grant Jr., G., Burgess, M., and Pla
the Sudan: A constructivist exploration. *Ch*

Brent, D. A., Perper, J. A., Moritz, G., Liotus
Schweers, J., and Roth, C. (1995). Posttraun
lescent suicide victims: Predisposing factors
American Academy of Child and Adolescer.

Brom, D., Kleber, R. J., and Defares, P. B. (1
traumatic stress disorders. *Journal of Cons*
607-612.

Brooks, B. and Siegel, P. M. (1996). *The scare*
matic events. New York: John Wiley and S

Bryant, R. A. and Harvey, A. G. (2000). *Acute*
ory, assessment, and treatment. Washingtor
sociation.

Canterbury, R. and Yule, W. (1999). Debriefin
(Ed.), *Post-traumatic stress disorders: Cc*
New York: John Wiley and Sons.

Carlson, E. B. and Rosser-Hogan, R. (1991).
stress, dissociation, and depression in Camb
Psychiatry, 148, 1548-1551.

Chaffin, M. (2000). What types of mental healt
maltreated children? In H. Dubowitz and I
child protection practice (pp. 409-413). The

Chard, K. M., Resick, P. A., and Wertz, J. J. (1
sault survivors. In B. H. Young and D. D.
post-traumatic stress disorder (pp. 35-51).

Chemtob, C. M., Tomas, S., Law, W., and
psychosocial intervention: A field study of
logical distress. *American Journal of Psych*

Chin, J. L. (1983). Diagnostic considerations
American Journal of Orthopsychiatry, 53, I

Cohen, J. A. and Mannarino, A. P. (1993). A t
preschoolers, *Journal of Interpersonal Viol*

Coll, C. T. G. and Meyer, E. C. (1993). The sociocultural context of infant development. In C. H. Zeanah Jr. (Ed.), *Handbook of infant mental health* (pp. 56-71). New York: Guilford Press.

Comas-Díaz, L. (1981). Puerto Rican espiritismo and psychotherapy. *American Journal of Orthopsychiatry, 51,* 637-645.

Cotton, C. R. and Range, L. M. (1990). Children's death concepts: Relationship to cognitive functioning, age, experience with death, fear of death, and hopelessness. *Journal of Clinical Child Psychology, 19,* 123-127.

Cowan, P. A. (1978). *Piaget with feeling: Cognitive, social, and emotional dimensions.* New York: Holt, Rinehart and Winston.

Crawford, J. B. (1992). Crisis management: You can make it if you plan. *Thrust for Educational Leadership, 22,* 29-32.

Crosby, J. and Van Soest, D. (1997). *Challenges of violence worldwide: An educational resource.* Washington, DC: NASW Press.

Cuddy Casey, M. and Orvaschel, H. (1997). Children's understanding of death in relation to child suicidality and homicidality. *Clinical Psychology Review, 17,* 33-45.

Cuéllar, I. and Paniagua, F. A. (Eds.) (2000). *Handbook of multicultural mental health: Assessment and treatment of diverse populations.* San Diego: Academic Press.

Dacey, J. S. and Travers, J. F. (1996). *Human development across the lifespan* (Third edition). Madison, WI: Brown and Benchmark.

Davidson, J. R. T. and Van der Kolk, B. A. (1996). The psychopharmacological treatment of posttraumatic stress disorder. In B. A. Van der Kolk, A. C. McFarlane, and L. Weisaeth (Eds.), *Traumatic stress: The effects of overwhelming experience on mind, body, and society* (pp. 510-525). New York: Guilford Press.

Dawes, A., Tredoux, C., and Feinstein, A. (1989). Political violence in South Africa: Some effects on children of the violent destruction of their community. *International Journal of Mental Health, 18,* 16-43.

Deblinger, E., McLeer, S. V., and Henry, D. (1990). Cognitive behavioral treatment for sexually abused children suffering post-traumatic stress: Preliminary findings. *Journal of the American Academy of Child and Adolescent Psychiatry, 29,* 747-752.

De Silva, P. and Samarasinghe, D. (1985). Behavior therapy in Sri Lanka. *Journal of Behavior Therapy and Experiential Psychiatry, 16,* 95-100.

DeVries, M. W. (1996). Trauma in cultural perspective. In B. A. Van der Kolk, A. C. McFarlane, and L. Weisaeth (Eds.), *Traumatic stress: The effects of overwhelming experience on mind, body, and society* (pp. 398-413). New York: Guilford Press.

Donnelly, C. L. and Amaya-Jackson, L. (2002). Post-traumatic stress disorder I—Children and adolescents: Epidemiology, diagnosis and treatment options. *Pediatric Drugs, 4,* 159-170.

Drell, M. J., Siegel, C. H., and Gaensbauer, T. J
der. In C. H. Zeanah Jr. (Ed.), *Handbook of*
New York: Guilford Press.

Dreman, S. and Cohen, E. (1990). Children of
grating individual and family treatment appr
psychiatry, 60, 204-209.

Dubowitz, H. and DePanfilis, D. (Eds.) (2000).
tice. Thousand Oaks, CA: Sage.

Dubrow, N. and Nader, K. (1999). Consultation
ing and honoring differences among cultures
Stamm (Eds.), *The series in trauma and lc*
issues in the treatment of trauma and loss
Mazel.

Dyregrov, A. (1997). The process in psycholo
matic Stress, 10, 589-605.

Eddleston, M., Rezvi, M. H., and Hawton, K.
Lanka: An overlooked tragedy in the develo
(International), 317, 133-135.

Ehrlich, E., Flexner, S. B., Carruth, G., and Ha
American dictionary. New York: Oxford Ur

Elmer, E. (1977). A follow-up study of trauma
279.

Erikson, E. H. (1950). *Childhood and society.* N
pany.

Figley, C. R. (Ed.) (1985). *Trauma and its wak*
traumatic stress disorder. New York: Brunn

Figley, C. R. (1989). *Helping traumatized fami*

Fingerhut, A., Cox, S., Warner, M., and Particip
tive Effort on Injury Statistics (1998). Intern
jury mortality: Findings from the ICE on i
<http://www.cdc.gov/nchs/data/ad/ad303.pd

Finsterbusch, K. and McKenna, G. (Eds.) (1996
controversial social issues (Ninth edition).
Benchmark.

Fivush, R., Haden, C., and Adam, S. (1995). Str
ers' personal narratives over time: Implicatic
of Experimental Child Psychology, 60, 32-5(

Flaskerud, J. H. and Liu, P. Y. (1991). Effects of
ethnicity and gender match on utilization an
Mental Health Journal, 27, 31-42.

Foa, E. B., Rothbaum, B. O., Riggs, D. S., and M
posttraumatic stress disorder in rape victims:

behavioral procedures and counseling. *Journal of Consulting and Clinical Psychology, 59,* 715-723.

Fox, J. A. and Zawitz, M. W. (1998). Homicide trends in the United States. United States Department of Justice. Bureau of Justice Statistics. Available online at <http://www.ojp.usdoj.gov/bjs>.

Freud, A. (1969). *The writings of Anna Freud: Research at the Hampstead Child-Therapy Clinic and other papers.* Volume V: *1956-1965.* New York: International Universities Press.

Friedman, S. (Ed.) (1997). *Cultural issues in the treatment of anxiety.* New York: Guilford Press.

Gaensbauer, T. J. and Siegel, C. H. (1995). Therapeutic approaches to posttraumatic stress disorder in infants and toddlers. *Infant Mental Health Journal, 16,* 293-305.

Galante, R. and Foa, D. (1986). An epidemiological study of psychic trauma and treatment effectiveness for children after a natural disaster. *Journal of the American Academy of Child Psychiatry, 25,* 357-363.

Garbarino, J. (1999). What children can tell us about living with violence. In M. Sugar (Ed.), *Trauma and Adolescence* (pp. 165-183). Madison, CT: International Universities Press.

Garbarino, J., Kostelny, K., and Dubrow, N. (1991). *No place to be a child. Growing up in a war zone.* Lexington, MA: Lexington Books.

George, C. and Main, M. (1979). Social interactions and young abused children: Approach, avoidance, and aggression. *Child Development, 50,* 306-319.

Gerber, L., Nguyen, Q., and Bounkeua, P. K. (1999). Working with Southeast Asian people who have migrated to the United States. In K. Nader, N. Dubrow, and B. H. Stamm (Eds.), *The series in trauma and loss: Honoring differences: Cultural issues in the treatment of trauma and loss* (pp. 98-116). Philadelphia: Brunner/Mazel.

Gerrity, E. T. and Solomon, S. D. (1996). The treatment of PTSD and related stress disorders: Current research and clinical knowledge. In A. J. Marsella, M. J. Friedman, E. T. Gerrity, and R. M. Scurfield (Eds.), *Ethnocultural aspects of posttraumatic stress disorder: Issues, research, and clinical applications* (pp. 87-104). Washington, DC: American Psychological Association.

Ghali, S. B. (1977). Culture sensitivity and the Puerto Rican client. *Social Casework, 58,* 459-468.

Giaconia, R. M., Reinherz, H. Z., Silverman, A. B., Pakiz, B., Frost, A. K., and Cohen, E. (1995). Traumas and posttraumatic stress disorder in a community population of older adolescents. *Journal of the American Academy of Child and Adolescent Psychiatry, 34,* 1369-1380.

Glod, C. A. and Teicher, M. H. (1996). Relationship between early abuse, posttraumatic stress disorder, and activity levels in prepubertal children. *Journal of the American Academy of Child and Adolescent Psychiatry, 35,* 1384-1393.

Goenjian, A., Karayan, I., Pynoos, R. S., Mina
    A. M., and Fairbanks, L. A. (1997). Outcon
    lescents after trauma. *American Journal of*
Goenjian, A. K., Pynoos, R. S., Steinberg, A.
    Karayan, I., Ghurabi, M., and Fairbanks, L
    in children after the 1988 earthquake in Arr
    emy of Child and Adolescent Psychiatry, 3
Goldstein, R. D., Wampler, N. S., and Wise, P
    tress symptoms of Bosnian children. *Pedic*
Goodman, G. S., Hirschman, J. E., Hepps, D
    memory for stressful events. *Merrill-Palm*
Gopaul-McNicol, S. and Brice-Baker, J. (199
    ment, treatment, and training. New York:
Green, A. (1993). Childhood sexual and physi
    phael (Eds.), *International handbook of tr*
    592). New York: Plenum Press.
Greenwald, R. (1999). *Eye movement desensiti*
    and adolescent psychotherapy. Northvale,
Han, A. L. and Vasquez, J. T. (2000). Group in
    minorities. In J. F. Aponte and J. Wohl (E
    cultural diversity (Second edition) (pp. 11(
Harkness, L. L. (1993). Transgenerational tra
    D. Meichenbaum, J. P. Wilson, and B.
    on stress and coping: International hand.
    (pp. 635-644). New York: Plenum Press.
Harmon, R. J. and Riggs, P.D. (1996). Clonidin
    preschool children. *Journal of the America*
    Psychiatry, 35, 1247-1249.
Higginbotham, H. N. (1984). *Third world chal*
    dation and mental health care. Honolulu: U
Hong, G. K., Garcia, M., and Soriano, M. (200
    paring mental health professionals for the
    F. A. Paniagua (Eds.), *Handbook of multicu*
    treatment of diverse populations (pp. 455-47
Husain, S. A., Nair, J., Holcomb, W., Reid, J. C
    Stress reactions of children and adolescent.
    can Journal of Psychiatry, 155, 1718-1719
James, B. (1994). Long-term treatment for ch
    M. B. Williams and J. F. Sommer Jr. (Eds.),
    (pp. 51-69). Westport, CT: Greenwood Pre
Jay, B. (1989). Managing a crisis in the school
    tin, 73, 14-18.

Jenkins, J. H. (1996). Culture, emotion, and PTSD. In A. J. Marsella, M. J. Fried-man, E. T. Gerrity, and R. M. Scurfield (Eds.), *Ethnocultural aspects of posttraumatic stress disorder: Issues, research, and clinical applications* (pp. 165-182). Washington, DC: American Psychological Association.

Joseph, S., Williams, R., and Yule, W. (1997). *Understanding post-traumatic stress: A psychosocial perspective on PTSD and treatment.* New York: John Wiley and Sons.

Kane, B. (1979). Children's concepts of death. *The Journal of Genetic Psychology, 134,* 141-153.

Kareem, J. (2000). The Nafsiyat Intercultural Therapy Centre: Ideas and experience in intercultural therapy. In J. Kareem and R. Littlewood (Eds.) *Intercultural therapy* (pp. 14-39). London: Blackwell Science.

Kareem, J. and Littlewood, R. (Eds.) (2000). *Intercultural therapy.* London: Blackwell Science.

Kinzie, J. D. (1993). Posttraumatic effects and their treatment among Southeast Asian refugees. In J. D. Meichenbaum, J. P. Wilson, and B. Raphael (Eds.), *The Plenum series on stress and coping: International handbook of traumatic stress syndromes* (pp. 311-320). New York: Plenum Press.

Kinzie, J. D. (2001). Psychotherapy for massively traumatised refugees: The therapist variable. *American Journal of Psychotherapy, 55,* 475-490.

Kinzie, J. D., Boehnlein, J. K., Leung, P. K., Moore, L. J., Riley, C., and Smith, D. (1990). The prevalence of posttraumatic stress disorder and its clinical significance among Southeast Asian refugees. *American Journal of Psychiatry, 147,* 913-917.

Kinzie, J. D., Sack, W. H., Angell, R. H., Manson, S., and Rath, B. (1986). The psychiatric effects of massive trauma on Cambodian children: I. The children. *Journal of the American Academy of Child Psychiatry, 25,* 370-376.

Kiser, L. J., Ackerman, B. J., Brown, E., Edwards, N. B., McColgan, E., Pugh, R., and Pruitt, D. B. (1988). Post-traumatic stress disorder in young children: A reaction to purported sexual abuse. *Journal of the American Academy of Child and Adolescent Psychiatry, 27,* 645-649.

Koss, J. D. (1987). Expectations and outcomes for patients given mental health care or spiritist healing in Puerto Rico. *American Journal of Psychiatry, 144,* 56-61.

Koss-Chioino, J. D. (2000). Traditional and folk approaches among ethnic minorities. In J. F. Aponte and J. Wohl (Eds.), *Psychological intervention and cultural diversity* (Second edition) (pp. 149-167). Boston: Allyn and Bacon.

Kroll, J., Habenicht, M., Mackenzie, T., Yang, M., Chan, S., Vang, T., Nguyen, T., Ly, M., Phommasouvanh, B., Nguyen, H., et al. (1989). Depression and posttraumatic stress disorder in Southeast Asian refugees. *American Journal of Psychiatry, 146,* 1592-1597.

Krystal, H. (1993). Beyond the DSM-lll-R: Therapeutic considerations in posttraumatic stress disorder. In D. Meichenbaum, J. P. Wilson, and B. Raphael

(Eds.), *The Plenum series on stress and co*
matic stress syndromes (pp. 841-854). Nev

Kübler-Ross, E. (1997). *On children and deatl*
and do cope with death. New York: Simor

Kurasaki, K. S., Sue, S., Chun, C., and Gee, K.
and treatment research. In J. F. Aponte and
vention and cultural diversity (Second editi
Bacon.

Landau, E. D., Epstein, S. L., and Stone, A.
through literature. Englewood Cliffs, NJ:

Laungani, P. (2001). Culture, cognition, and t
J. F. Schumaker and T. Ward (Eds.), *Cult*
(pp. 119-145). Westport, CT: Praeger.

Lee, E. (1988). Cultural factors in working v
cents. *Journal of Adolescence, 11,* 167-17ᶜ

Leff, J. (1981). *Psychiatry around the globe: A*
cel Dekker.

Lerner, M., Volpe, J., and Lindell, B. (2003).
Empowering educators during traumatic
Academy of Experts in Traumatic Stress.

Lester, D. (1997). Suicide in an international
ening Behavior, 27, 104-111.

Lin, K., Inui, T., Kleinman, A.M., and Womac
minants of the help-seeking behavior of patᶦ
of Nervous and Mental Disease, 170, 78-8ᴉ

Loff, B. and Cordner, S. (1998). Suicide in A
633-634.

Lonigan, C.J., Shannon, M. P., Taylor, C. M
(1994). Children exposed to disaster: II.
post-traumatic symptomatology. *Journal o*
Adolescent Psychology, 33, 94-105.

Machel, G. (1996). The impact of armed confl
Nations General Assembly. Available on
ga/docs/51/plenary/A51-306.EN>.

Macksoud, M. S., Dyregrov, A., and Raundale
ences and their effects on children. In D. Mɛ
phael (Eds.), *The Plenum series on stress ar*
traumatic stress syndromes (pp. 625-634).

Malmquist, C. P. (1986). Children who witnes
pects. *Journal of the American Academy of*

March, J. S., Amaya-Jackson, L., and Murray,
psychotherapy for children and adolescents
nal of the American Academy of Child and A

Marcos, L. R. (1979). Effects of interpreters on the evaluation of psychopathology in non-English-speaking patients. *American Journal of Psychiatry, 136,* 171-174.

Marks, I., Lovell, K., Noshirvani, H., Livanou, M., and Thrasher, S. (1998). Treatment of posttraumatic stress disorder by exposure and/or cognitive restructuring. *Archives of General Psychiatry, 55,* 317-325.

Marsella, A. J., Friedman, M. J., Gerrity, E. T., and Scurfield, R. M. (1996). Ethnocultural aspects of PTSD: Some closing thoughts. In A. J. Marsella, M. J. Friedman, E. T. Gerrity, and R. M. Scurfield (Eds.), *Ethnocultural aspects of posttraumatic stress disorder: Issues, research, and clinical applications* (pp. 529-538). Washington, DC: American Psychological Association.

Marshall, R. D., Yehuda, R., and Bone, S. (2000). Trauma-focused psychodynamic psychotherapy for individuals with posttraumatic stress symptoms. In D. Meichenbaum, A. Y. Shalev, R. Yehuda, and A. C. McFarlane (Eds.), *The Plenum series on stress and coping: International handbook of human response to trauma* (pp. 337-346). New York: Kluwer Academic/Plenum.

Martin, P. and Midgley, E. (2003). Immigration: Shaping and reshaping America. *Population Bulletin, 58,* 1-47.

Martín-Baró, I. (1989). Political violence and war as causes of psychosocial trauma in El Salvador. *International Journal of Mental Health, 18,* 3-20.

Mbiti, J. S. (1990). *African religions and philosophy* (Second edition). Oxford, England: Heinemann Educational Books.

McFarlane, A. C. (1987). Posttraumatic phenomena in a longitudinal study of children following a natural disaster. *Journal of the American Academy of Child and Adolescent Psychiatry, 26,* 764-769.

McFarlane, A. C. and Van der Kolk, B. A. (1996). Trauma and its challenge to society. In B. A. Van der Kolk, A. C. McFarlane, and L. Weisaeth (Eds.), *Traumatic stress: The effects of overwhelming experience on mind, body, and society* (pp. 24-46). New York: Guilford Press.

Meadows, E. A. and Foa, E. B. (2000). Cognitive behavioral treatment for PTSD. In D. Meichenbaum, A. Y. Shalev, R. Yehuda, and A. C. McFarlane (Eds.), *The Plenum series on stress and coping: International handbook of human response to trauma* (pp. 337-346). New York: Kluwer Academic/Plenum.

Meichenbaum, D., Shalev, A. Y., Yehuda, R., and McFarlane, A. C. (Eds.) (2000). *The Plenum series on stress and coping: International handbook of human response to trauma.* New York: Kluwer Academic/Plenum.

Meichenbaum, D., Wilson, J. P., and Raphael, B. (Eds.) (1993). *The Plenum series on stress and coping: International handbook of traumatic stress syndromes.* New York: Plenum Press.

Melville, M. B. and Lykes, M. B. (1992). Guatemalan Indian children and the sociocultural effects of government sponsored terrorism. *Social Science and Medicine, 34,* 533-548.

Michel, L. and Herbeck, D. (2001). *American*
Oklahoma City bombing. New York: Harpe

Mitchell, J. T. (1983). When disaster strikes: T
process. *Journal of Emergency Medical Se*

Mitchell, J. T. and Dyregrov, A. (1993). Trau
emergency personnel: Prevention and inter
phael (Eds.), *International handbook of tr*
914). New York: Plenum Press.

Monahon, C. (1993). *Children and trauma: A*
heal. New York: Lexington Books.

Moriarty, A., Maeyama, R. G., and Fitzgerald,
crisis management. *NAASP Bulletin, 77, 17*

Mullins, W. C. (1997). *A sourcebook on dome*
analysis of issues, organizations, tactics, and
field, IL: Charles C. Thomas.

Nader, K., Dubrow, N., and Stamm, B. H. (Ed
loss: Honoring differences: Cultural issues
Philadelphia: Brunner/Mazel.

Nader, K., Pynoos, R., Fairbanks, L., and Frede
actions one year after a sniper attack at their
atry, 147, 1526-1530.

National Center for Education Statistics (NCE
problems in U.S. public schools: 1996-97.
gov/pubs98/violence/index.html>. March.

National Center for Education Statistics (NCES
and safety 2002. Available online at <ht
index.asp>.

National Center for Injury Prevention and C
causes of death, United States 2001. Availab
cgi-bin/broker.exe>.

National Clearinghouse on Child Abuse and Ne
What is child maltreatment? Available
nccanchpubs/factsheets/whatis.htm>.

National Climatic Data Center (NCDC), Nati
ministration (NOAA) (1999). Climate of 19
able online at <http://www.ncdc.noaa.gov
html>. June 8.

National Climatic Data Center (NCDC), Nati
ministration (NOAA) (n.d.). Flooding in Ch
at <http://www.ncdc.noaa.gov/ol/reports/ch

National Climatic Data Center (NCDC), Nati
ministration (NOAA) (n.d.). Mitch: The dea
Available online at <http://www.ncdc.noaa

National Highway Traffic Safety Administration (NHTSA), Department of Transportation (DOT) (n.d.). Traffic safety facts 2001. Available online at <http://www.nrd.nhtsa.dot.gov/>.

National Hurricane Center (NHC) (1999). Preliminary report. Hurricane Georges 15 September-01 October 1998. Available online at <http://www.nhc.noaa.gov/1998 georges.html>. January 5.

National Oceanic and Atmospheric Administration (NOAA) (1998). Year-end tip sheet: Top weather and NOAA/national weather stories. Available online at <http://www.publicaffairs.noaa.gov/weather98/>.

National Oceanic and Atmospheric Administration (NOAA), National Climatic Data Center (NCDC) (n.d.). California flooding and Florida tornadoes. Available online at <http://www.ncdc.noaa.gov/ol/reports/febstorm/february98storms.html#Calif>.

Newman, C. J. (1976). Children of disaster: Clinical observations at Buffalo Creek. *American Journal of Psychiatry, 133,* 306-312.

O'Brien, L. S. (1998). *Traumatic events and mental health.* Cambridge, UK: Cambridge University Press.

O'Hare, W. P. (1992). America's minorities: The demographics of diversity. *Population Bulletin, 47,* 1-47.

Orbach, I. and Glaubman, H. (1979). Children's perception of death as a defensive process. *Journal of Abnormal Psychology, 88,* 671-674.

Papalia, D. E. and Olds, S. W. (1993). *A child's world: Infancy through adolescence* (Sixth edition). New York: McGraw-Hill.

Parson, E. R. (1985). Ethnicity and traumatic stress: The intersecting point in psychotherapy. In C. R. Figley (Ed.), *Trauma and its wake: The study and treatment of post-traumatic stress disorder* (pp. 314-338). New York: Brunner/Mazel.

Parson, E. R. (1997). Posttraumatic child therapy (P-TCT) assessment and treatment factors in clinical work with inner-city children exposed to catastrophic community violence. *Journal of Interpersonal Violence, 12,* 172-194.

Peddle, N., Monteiro, C., Guluma, V., and Macaulay, T. E. A. (1999). Trauma, loss, and resilience in Africa: A psychosocial community based approach to culturally sensitive healing. In K. Nader, N. Dubrow, and B. H. Stamm (Eds.), *The series in trauma and loss: Honoring differences: Cultural issues in the treatment of trauma and loss* (pp. 121-150). Philadelphia: Brunner/Mazel.

Pernice, R. and Brook, J. (1994). Relationship of migrant status (refugee or immigrant) to mental health. *The International Journal of Social Psychiatry, 40,* 177-188.

Perren-Klinger, G. (2000). The integration of traumatic experiences: Culture and resources. In J. M. Violanti, D. Paton, and C. Dunning (Eds.), *Posttraumatic stress intervention: Challenges, issues, and perspectives* (pp. 43-62). Springfield, IL: Charles C. Thomas.

Peterson, K. C., Prout, M. F., and Schwarz, R.A. (1991). *Post-traumatic stress disorder: A clinician's guide.* New York: Plenum Press.

Pfefferbaum, B. (1997). Posttraumatic stress d
  past 10 years. *Journal of the American Acad*
  atry, 36, 1503-1511.

Pfefferbaum, B., Nixon, S. J., Krug, R. S., Tivis
  Pynoos, R. S., Foy, D., and Gurwitch, R. H. (
  middle and high school students following
  American Journal of Psychiatry, 156, 1069-

Pfefferbaum, B., Nixon, S. J., and Tucker, P.
  sponses in bereaved children after the Okla
  American Academy of Child and Adolescen

Phinney, J. S. (1996). When we talk about A
  mean? *American Psychologist, 51,* 918-927

Podolefsky, A. and Brown, P. J. (1997). *Applyi*
  ductory reader (Third edition). Mountain V

Pollard, K. M. and O'Hare, W. P. (1999). Am
  Population Bulletin, 54, p. 2.

Porter, R. Y. (2000). Understanding and treat
  Aponte and J. Wohl (Eds.), *Psychological*
  (Second edition) (pp. 167-183). Boston: Al

Potter, L. (1997). Getting the media on our side

Protacio-Marcelino, E. (1989). Children of po
  Sources of stress and coping patterns. *Inter.*
  18, 71-86.

Pruett, K. D. (1979). Home treatment for two in
  murder. *Journal of the American Academy c*

Pynoos, R. S., and Eth, S. (1985a). Children tra
  sonal violence: Homicide, rape, or suicide b
  (Eds.), *Post-traumatic stress disorder in chi*
  American Psychiatric Press.

Pynoos, R. and Eth, S. (1985b). Developmenta
  childhood. In C. R. Figley (Ed.), *Trauma an*
  of post-traumatic stress disorder (pp. 36-53

Pynoos, R. S., Frederick, C., Nader, K., Arroyo
  F., and Fairbanks, L. (1987). Life threat and
  children. *Archives of General Psychiatry, 44*

Pynoos, R. S. and Nader, K. (1988). Children
  their mothers. *Journal of the American Aca*
  chiatry, 27, 567-572.

Pynoos, R. S. and Nader, K. (1989). Case study
  to violence. *Journal of the American Academ*
  try, 28, 236-241.

Pynoos, R. S. and Nader, K. (1993). Issues in the
  children and adolescents. In D. Meichenba

(Eds.), *The Plenum series on stress and coping: International handbook of traumatic stress syndromes: International handbook of traumatic stress syndromes* (pp. 535-550). New York: Plenum Press.

Reilly, T. P., Hasazi, J. E., and Bond, L. A. (1983). Children's conceptions of death and personal mortality. *Journal of Pediatric Psychology, 8,* 21-31.

Richards, D. and Lovell, K. (1999). Behavioural and cognitive behavioural interventions in the treatment of PTSD. In W. Yule (Ed.), *Post-traumatic stress disorders: Concepts and therapy* (pp. 239-266). New York: John Wiley and Sons.

Rothbaum, B. O. and Schwartz, A. C. (2002). Exposure therapy for posttraumatic stress disorder. *American Journal of Psychotherapy, 56,* 59-74.

Roy, C. A. and Russell, R. C. (2000). Case study: Possible traumatic stress disorder in an infant with cancer. *Journal of the American Academy of Child and Adolescent Psychiatry, 39,* 257-260.

Ruiz, P. and Langrod, J. (1976). Psychiatry and folk healing: A dichotomy? *American Journal of Psychiatry, 133,* 95-97.

Russoniello, C. V., Skalko, T. K., O'Brien, K., McGhee, S. A., Bingham-Alexander, D., and Beatley, J. (2002). Childhood posttraumatic stress disorder and efforts to cope after Hurricane Floyd. *Behavioral Medicine, 28,* 61-71.

Sack, W. H., Angell, R. H., Kinzie, J. D., and Rath, B. (1986). The psychiatric effects of massive trauma on Cambodian children: II. The family, the home, and the school. *Journal of the American Academy of Child Psychiatry, 25,* 377-383.

Saigh, P. A., Yule, W., and Inamdar, S. C. (1996). Imaginal flooding of traumatized children and adolescents. *Journal of School Psychology, 34,* 163-183.

Saylor, C. F., Swenson, C. C., and Powell, P. (1992). Hurricane Hugo blows down the broccoli: Preschoolers' post-disaster play and adjustment. *Child Psychiatry and Human Development, 22,* 139-149.

Schachter, R. and McCauley, C. S. (1988). *When your child is afraid: Understanding the normal fears of childhood from birth through adolescence and helping overcome them.* New York: Simon and Schuster.

Scheeringa, M. S. and Zeanah. C. H. (1995). Symptom expression and trauma variables in children under 48 months of age. *Infant Mental Health Journal, 16,* 259-269.

Scheeringa, M. S., Zeanah, C. H., Drell, M. J., and Larrieu, J. A. (1995). Two approaches to the diagnosis of posttraumatic stress disorder in infancy and early childhood. *Journal of the American Academy of Child and Adolescent Psychiatry, 34,* 191-200.

Schumaker, J. F. and Ward, T. (Eds.) (2001). *Cultural cognition and psychopathology.* Westport, CT: Praeger.

Schuster, M. A., Stein, B. D., Jaycox, L. H., Collins, L. R., Marshall, G. W., Elliott, M. N., Zhou, A. J., Kanouse, D. E., Morrison, J. L., and Berry, S. H. (2001). A national survey of stress reactions after the September 11, 2001, terrorist attacks. *New England Journal of Medicine, 345,* 1507-1512.

Schwarz, E. D. and Kowalski, J. M. (1991). M: and adults after a school shooting. *Journa and Adolescent Psychiatry, 30,* 936-944.

Scurfield, R. M. (1985). Post-trauma stress a and formulating. In C. R. Figley (Ed.), *T treatment of post-traumatic stress disordε ner/Mazel.

Shannon, M. P., Lonigan, C. J., Finch, A. J. Jr exposed to disaster: I. Epidemiology of po: profiles. *Journal of the American Academy 33,* 80-93.

Shapiro, F. (1989). Eye movement desensit traumatic stress disorder. *Journal of Behavι atry, 20,* 211-217.

Shaw, J. A., Applegate, B., Tanner, S., Perez, and Lahey, B. L. (1995). Psychological eff mentary school population. *Journal of the ∤ lescent Psychiatry, 34,* 1185-1192.

Silove, D. and Schweitzer, R. (1993). Aparthei in conflict. In J. P. Wilson and B. Raphaε *traumatic stress syndromes* (pp. 645-650).

Silver, S. M. and Rogers, S. (2002). *Light in tι treatment of war and terrorism survivors.*] pany.

Simon, J. D. (2001). *The terrorist trap: Ameri ond edition).* Bloomington: Indiana Univer

Simpson, M. A. (1993). Bitter waters: Effects and oppression. In D. Meichenbaum, J. P. *Plenum series on stress and coping: Internε syndromes* (pp. 601-624). New York: Plen

Somé, M. P. (1998). *The healing wisdom of ∤ nature, ritual, and community.* New York:

Sue, S., Fujino, D. C., Li-tze, H., Takeuchi, D. munity mental health services for ethnic m responsiveness hypothesis. *Journal of Con 533-540.

Sue, S. and Zane, N. (1987). The role of cultuι therapy: A critique and reformulation. *Amε

Sugar, M. (1988). A preschooler in a disaster. *42,* 619-629.

Sugar, M. (Ed.) (1999). *Trauma and adolescεr versities Press.

Swain, H. (1979). Childhood views of death. ∤

Swartz, L. (1998). *Culture and mental health: A southern African view*. Cape Town: Oxford University Press.

Tanaka-Matsumi, J., Seiden, D. Y., and Lam, K. N. (2001). Translating cultural observations into psychotherapy: A functional approach. In J. F. Schumaker and T. Ward (Eds.), *Cultural cognition and psychopathology* (pp. 193-213). Madison, CT: Praeger.

Tarrier, N., Pilgrim, H., Sommerfield, S., Faragher, B., Reynolds, M., Graham, E., and Barrowclough, C. (1999). A randomized trial of cognitive therapy and imaginal exposure in the treatment of chronic posttraumatic stress disorder. *Journal of Consulting and Clinical Psychology, 67,* 13-18.

Terr, L. C. (1981a). "Forbidden games": Post-traumatic child's play. *Journal of the American Academy of Child Psychiatry, 20,* 741-760.

Terr, L. C. (1981b). Psychic trauma in children: Observations following the Chowchilla school-bus kidnapping. *American Journal of Psychiatry, 138,* 15-19.

Terr, L. C. (1983). Chowchilla revisited: The effects of psychic trauma four years after a school-bus kidnapping. *American Journal of Psychiatry, 140,* 1543-1550.

Terr, L. (1990). *Too scared to cry: Psychic trauma in childhood* (First edition). New York: Harper and Row.

Terr, L. C. (1991). Childhood traumas: An outline and overview. *American Journal of Psychiatry, 148,* 10-20.

Terr, L. C., Bloch, D. A., Michel, B. A., Shi, H., Reinhardt, J. A., and Metayer, S. (1996). Children's memories in the wake of *Challenger. American Journal of Psychiatry, 153,* 618-625.

Tharp, R. G. (1991). Cultural diversity and treatment of children. *Journal of Consulting and Clinical Psychology, 59,* 799-812.

Thomas, D. (1993). Crisis communication. *Thrust for Educational Leadership, 23,* 17-20.

Toupin, E. S. W. A. (1980). Counseling Asians: Psychotherapy in the context of racism and Asian-American history. *American Journal of Orthopsychiatry, 50,* 76-88.

Trotter, R. T. II and Chavira, J. A. (1997). *Curanderismo: Mexican American folk healing* (Second edition). Athens: The University of Georgia Press.

Tseng, W.S., Di, X., Ebata, K., Hsu, J., and Yuhua, C. (1986). Diagnostic pattern for neurosis in China, Japan, and the United States. *American Journal of Psychiatry, 143,* 1010-1014.

Tully, M. A. (1999). Lifting our voices: African-American cultural responses to trauma and loss. In K. Nader, N. Dubrow, and B. H. Stamm (Eds.), *The series in trauma and loss: Honoring differences: Cultural issues in the treatment of trauma and loss* (pp. 23-49). Philadelphia: Brunner/Mazel.

United Nations Children's Fund (UNICEF) (1993). *The state of the world's children 1994.* New York: Oxford University Press for UNICEF.

United Nations Children's Fund (UNICEF) (1995). *The state of the world's children 1996.* New York: Oxford University Press for UNICEF.

United Nations Children's Fund (UNICEF) (
   dren 1997. New York: Oxford University

United Nations Children's Fund (UNICEF) (
   dren 2001. New York: Oxford University

United States Department of Health and H
   Children and Families, Children's Burea
   Available online at <http://nccanch.acf.hh

United States Fire Administration, Federal Em
   Curious kids set fires: A fact sheet for te
   <http://www.usfa.fema.gov/public/curious

United States Fire Administration, Federal Em
   Facts on fire. Available online at <http://ww

United States Fire Administration, Federal Em
   The overall fire picture—2002. Available c
   inside-usfa/nfdc-data.shtm>.

United States Geological Survey (USGS), Nat
   (NEIC) (n.d.). Earthquake facts and sta
   wwwneic.cr.usgs.gov/neis/eqlists/eqstats.h

U.S. Department of Justice, Bureau of Justice
   Violent offenders and their victims. Availabl
   bjs/abstract/cvvoatv.htm>.

U.S. Department of State (2001). The year in r
   2000. Available online at <http://www.state

U.S. Department of State (2004). Patterns of
   <http://www.state.gov/s/ct/rls/pgtrpt/2003/

Valsiner, J. (Ed.) (1989). *Child development i*
   and Huber.

Van der Kolk, B. A. (1996). The complexity of
   stimulus discrimination, and characterolog
   Kolk, A. C. McFarlane, and L. Weisaeth (E
   overwhelming experience on mind, body, a
   Guilford Press.

Van der Kolk, B. A., McFarlane, A. C., and W
   stress: The effects of overwhelming experie
   York: Guilford Press.

Van der Veer, G. (1998). *Counselling and th*
   trauma: Psychological problems of victi
   (Second edition). New York: John Wiley a

Vélez-Ibáñez, C. G. and Parra, C. G. (1999).
   concerning mental health concepts and pra
   west United States with reference to o
   N. Dubrow, and B. H. Stamm (Eds.), *The*

differences: Cultural issues in the treatment of trauma and loss (pp. 76-98). Philadelphia: Brunner/Mazel.

Watts, J. (1998). Suicide rate rises as South Korea's economy falters. *Lancet, 352,* 1365.

Wayne, G. (1992). Polishing the public's perception. *Thrust for Educational Leadership, 22,* 34-39.

Westermeyer, J. (1985). Psychiatric diagnosis across cultural boundaries. *American Journal of Psychiatry, 142,* 798-805.

Westermeyer, J. (1990). Working with an interpreter in psychiatric assessment and treatment. *Journal of Nervous and Mental Disorders, 178,* 745-749.

Williams, J. K. (1993). Giving (and getting) good press. *Thrust for Educational Leadership, 23,* 28-31.

Williams, L. M. and Banyard, V. L. (Eds.) (1998). *Trauma and memory.* Thousand Oaks, CA: Sage Publications.

Williams, M. B. (1994). Intervention with child victims of trauma in the school setting. In M. B. Williams and J. F. Sommer Jr. (Eds.), *Handbook of post-traumatic therapy* (pp. 69-78).Westport, CT: Greenwood Press.

Williams, M. B. and Sommer, J. F. Jr. (Eds.) (1994). *Handbook of post-traumatic therapy.* Westport, CT: Greenwood Press.

Wilson, M. N., Kohn, L. P., and Lee, T. S. (2000). Cultural relativistic approach toward ethnic minorities in family therapy. In J. F. Aponte and J. Wohl (Eds.), *Psychological intervention and cultural diversity* (Second edition) (pp. 92-110). Boston: Allyn and Bacon.

Wilson-Oyelaran, E. B. (1989). Toward contextual sensitivity in developmental psychology: A Nigerian perspective. In J. Valsiner (Ed.), *Child development in cultural context* (pp. 51-67). Toronto: Hogrefe and Huber.

Wolfe, V. V., Gentile, C., and Wolfe, D. A. (1989). The impact of sexual abuse on children: A PTSD formulation. *Behavior Therapy, 20,* 215-228.

World Congress Against the Commercial Sexual Exploitation of Children (n.d.). Fact sheet. Available online at <http://www.usis.usemb.se/children/csec/factsheets.hem>.

World Meteorological Organization (WMO), United Nations (n.d.). WMO: For a safer world. Available online at <gopher://gopher.un.org/00/conf/wssd/pc-3/bkg/950227121914.txt>.

Young, B. H. and Blake, D. D. (Eds.) (1999). *Group treatments for post-traumatic stress disorder.* Philadelphia: Brunner/Mazel.

Yule, W. (Ed.) (1999). *Post-traumatic stress disorders: Concepts and therapy.* New York: John Wiley and Sons.

Yule, W., Perrin, S., and Smith, P. (1999). Post-traumatic disorders in children and adolescents. In W. Yule (Ed.), *Post-traumatic stress disorders: Concepts and therapy* (pp. 25-50). New York: John Wiley and Sons.

Yule, W., Udwin, O., and Murdoch, K. (1990). The "Jupiter" sinking: Effects on children's fears, depression and anxiety. *Journal of Child Psychology and Psychiatry, 31,* 1051-1061.

Zahr, L. K. (1996). Effects of war on the beha̅
    Influence of home environment and famil̅
    Orthopsychiatry, 66, 401-408.
Zeanah, C. H. Jr. (Ed.) (1993). *Handbook c̅*
    Guilford Press.
Živčić, I. (1993). Emotional reactions of childr̅
    the American Academy of Child and Adole̅

Index

Page numbers followed by the letter "b" indicate boxed text.

EFFECTS OF AND INTERVENTIONS FOR CHILDHOOD TRAUMA FROM INFANCY THROUGH ADOLESCENCE: PAIN UNSPEAKABLE by Sandra B. Hutchison (2005). "Insightful, provocative, informative, and resourceful. This book needs to be in the hands of all professionals working with children, preparting to work with children, or considering work with children. It illustrates the many faces of trauma and illuminates the many responses of children to trauma." *Osofo Calvin Banks, MDiv, Founder and Facilitator, Sesa Woruban Center for Spiritual Development; Certified Supervisor, Association for Clinical and Pastoral Education, Inc.*

SCHIZOPHRENIA: INNOVATIONS IN DIAGNOSIS AND TREATMENT by Colin A. Ross. (2004). "Well-documented and clearly explained ... has hugely significant implications for our diagnostic system and for how severely disturbed people are understood and treated." *John Read, PhD, Editor,* Models of Madness: Psychological, Social, and Biological Approaches to Schizophrenia; *Director of Clinical Psychology, The University of Auckland, New Zealand*

REBUILDING ATTACHMENTS WITH TRAUMATIZED CHILDREN: HEALING FROM LOSSES, VIOLENCE, ABUSE, AND NEGLECT by Richard Kagan. "Dr. Richard Kagan, a recognized expert in working with traumatized children, has written a truly impressive book. Not only does the book contain a wealth of information for understanding the complex issues faced by traumatized youngsters, but it also offers specific interventions that can be used to help these children and their caregivers become more hopeful and resilient. . . . I am certain that this book will be read and reread by professionals engaged in improving the lives of at-risk youth." *Robert Brooks, PhD, Faculty, Harvard Medical School and author of* Raising Resilient Children *and* The Power of Resilience

PSYCHOLOGICAL TRAUMA AND THE DEVELOPING BRAIN: NEUROLOGICALLY BASED INTERVENTIONS FOR TROUBLED CHILDREN by Phyllis T. Stien and Joshua C. Kendall. (2003). "Stien and Kendall provide us with a great service. In this clearly written and important book, they synthesize a wealth of crucial information that links childhood trauma to brain abnormalities and subsequent mental illness. Equally important, they show us how the trauma also affects the child's social and intellectual development. I recommend this book to all clinicians and administrators." *Charles L. Whitfield, MD, Author of* The Truth About Depression *and* The Truth About Mental Illness

CHILD MALTREATMENT RISK ASSESSMENTS: AN EVALUATION GUIDE by Sue Righthand, Bruce Kerr, and Kerry Drach. (2003). "This book is essential reading for clinicians and forensic examiners who see cases involving issues related to child maltreatment. The authors have compiled an impressive critical survey of the relevant research on child maltreatment. Their material is well organized into sections on definitions, impact, risk assessment, and risk management. This book represents a giant step toward promoting evidence-based evaluations, treatment, and testimony." *Diane H. Schetky, MD, Professor of Psychiatry, University of Vermont College of Medicine*

SIMPLE AND COMPLEX POST-TRAUMA'
EGIES FOR COMPREHENSIVE TREATMEN
Mary Beth Williams and John F. Sommer Jr. (2002)
treating survivors of traumatic events, this volume ｢
even the experienced clinician to master the manage
Keane, PhD, Chief, Psychology Service, VA Bostor
Chair of Research in Psychiatry, Boston University

FOR LOVE OF COUNTRY: CONFRONTING Ι
IN THE U.S. MILITARY by T. S. Nelson. (2002).
that the absence of current media attention doesn't m
decisive action by military leadership at all levels
tization; and that the failure to do so is, as Nelson pu
positive leadership at all levels to stop violent indiviｃ
able." *Chris Lombardi, Correspondent, Women's E·*

THE INSIDERS: A MAN'S RECOVERY FROM
by Robert Blackburn Knight. (2002). "An importaʼ
about healing from childhood sexual abuse by allov
one man's history and journey of recovery." *Amy P.*
founder, Survivors Healing Center, Santa Cruz, Caｆ

WE ARE NOT ALONE: A GUIDEBOOK FOР
PARENTS SUPPORTING ADOLESCENT VIᏟ
Christine Angelica. (2002). "Encourages victims aｒ
tem in an effort to heal from their victimization, seeʼ
for their crimes. An exceedingly vital training tool."
Assistance Program and Children's Advocacy Cent
fice, Boston

WE ARE NOT ALONE: A TEENAGE GIRL'S Ι
FROM DISCLOSURE THROUGH PROSECʟ
Christine Angelica. (2002). "A valuable resource fｅ
and their parents. With compassion and eloquent pｒ
criminal justice system—from disclosure to final oｕ
Research Associate, Family Research Laboratory, ｌ

WE ARE NOT ALONE: A TEENAGE BOY'S
SEXUAL ABUSE FROM DISCLOSURE THRO
MENT by Jade Christine Angelica. (2002). "Inspirｅ
answer their questions, calm their fears, and protect
which is often not designed to respond to them in a lｅ
JD, Assistant District Attorney, Middlesex, Massach

GROWING FREE: A MANUAL FOR SURVIVᏟ
Wendy Susan Deaton and Michael Hertica. (2001). "
is scared and starting to think about what it would
friends and relatives of a person in a domestic violenｅ
leen Friend, LCSW, Field Work Consultant, UCLA ﹐
Public Policy & Social Research

A THERAPIST'S GUIDE TO GROWING FREE: A MANUAL FOR SURVIVORS OF DOMESTIC VIOLENCE by Wendy Susan Deaton and Michael Hertica. (2001). "An excellent synopsis of the theories and research behind the manual." *Beatrice Crofts Yorker, RN, JD, Professor of Nursing, Georgia State University, Decatur*

PATTERNS OF CHILD ABUSE: HOW DYSFUNCTIONAL TRANSACTIONS ARE REPLICATED IN INDIVIDUALS, FAMILIES, AND THE CHILD WELFARE SYSTEM by Michael Karson. (2001). "No one interested in what may well be the major public health epidemic of our time in terms of its long-term consequences for our society can afford to pass up the opportunity to read this enlightening work." *Howard Wolowitz, PhD, Professor Emeritus, Psychology Department, University of Michigan, Ann Arbor*

IDENTIFYING CHILD MOLESTERS: PREVENTING CHILD SEXUAL ABUSE BY RECOGNIZING THE PATTERNS OF THE OFFENDERS by Carla van Dam. (2000). "The definitive work on the subject. . . . Provides parents and others with the tools to recognize when and how to intervene." *Roger W. Wolfe, MA, Co-Director, N. W. Treatment Associates, Seattle, Washington*

POLITICAL VIOLENCE AND THE PALESTINIAN FAMILY: IMPLICATIONS FOR MENTAL HEALTH AND WELL-BEING by Vivian Khamis. (2000). "A valuable book . . . a pioneering work that fills a glaring gap in the study of Palestinian society." *Elia Zureik, Professor of Sociology, Queens University, Kingston, Ontario, Canada*

STOPPING THE VIOLENCE: A GROUP MODEL TO CHANGE MEN'S ABUSIVE ATTITUDES AND BEHAVIORS by David J. Decker. (1999). "A concise and thorough manual to assist clinicians in learning the causes and dynamics of domestic violence." *Joanne Kittel, MSW, LICSW, Yachats, Oregon*

STOPPING THE VIOLENCE: A GROUP MODEL TO CHANGE MEN'S ABUSIVE ATTITUDES AND BEHAVIORS, THE CLIENT WORKBOOK by David J. Decker. (1999).

BREAKING THE SILENCE: GROUP THERAPY FOR CHILDHOOD SEXUAL ABUSE, A PRACTITIONER'S MANUAL by Judith A. Margolin. (1999). "This book is an extremely valuable and well-written resource for all therapists working with adult survivors of child sexual abuse." *Esther Deblinger, PhD, Associate Professor of Clinical Psychiatry, University of Medicine and Dentistry of New Jersey School of Osteopathic Medicine*

"I NEVER TOLD ANYONE THIS BEFORE": MANAGING THE INITIAL DISCLOSURE OF SEXUAL ABUSE RE-COLLECTIONS by Janice A. Gasker. (1999). "Discusses the elements needed to create a safe, therapeutic environment and offers the practitioner a number of useful strategies for responding appropriately to client disclosure." *Roberta G. Sands, PhD, Associate Professor, University of Pennsylvania School of Social Work*

FROM SURVIVING TO THRIVING: A THERAPIST'S GUIDE TO STAGE II RECOVERY FOR SURVIVORS OF CHILDHOOD ABUSE by Mary Bratton. (1999). "A must read for all, including survivors. Bratton takes a lifelong debilitating disorder and unravels its intricacies in concise, succinct, and understandable language." *Phillip A. Whitner, PhD, Sr. Staff Counselor, University Counseling Center, The University of Toledo, Ohio*

SIBLING ABUSE TRAUMA: ASSESSMENT AND INTERVENTION STRATEGIES FOR CHILDREN, FAMILIES, AND ADULTS by John V. Caffaro and Allison Conn-Caffaro. (1998). "One area that has almost consistently been ignored in the research and writing on child maltreatment is the area of sibling abuse. This book is a welcome and required addition to the developing literature on abuse." *Judith L. Alpert, PhD, Professor of Applied Psychology, New York University*

Printed and bound by CPI Group (UK) Ltd, Croydon, CR0 4YY

17/10/2024

01775687-0002